LOW POTASSIUM DIET COOKBOOK, FOOD LIST, AND MEAL PLAN FOR SENIORS

Delicious Recipes with Low Sodium, Phosphorus, and Potassium for a Healthier, Happier Life

Meadows Julia McIntyre

Copyright © 2024 Meadows Julia McIntyre

All Rights Are Reserved

The content in this book may not be reproduced, duplicated, or transferred without the express written permission of the author or publisher. Under no circumstances will the publisher or author be held liable or legally responsible for any losses, expenditures, or damages incurred directly or indirectly as a consequence of the information included in this book.

Legal Remarks

Copyright protection applies to this publication. It is only intended for personal use. No piece of this work may be modified, distributed, sold, quoted, or paraphrased without the author's or publisher's consent.

Disclaimer Statement

Please keep in mind that the contents of this booklet are meant for educational and recreational purposes. Every effort has been made to offer accurate, up-to-date, reliable, and thorough information. There are, however, no stated or implied assurances of any kind. Readers understand that the author is providing competent counsel. The content in this book originates from several sources. Please seek the opinion of a competent professional before using any of the tactics outlined in this book. By reading this book, the reader agrees that the author will not be held accountable for any direct or indirect damages resulting from the use of the information contained therein, including, but not limited to, errors, omissions, or inaccuracies.

Table of Contents

INTRODUCTION 1

Chapter One: 4

IMPORTANCE OF POTASSIUM REGULATION IN SENIORS 4

Chapter Two: 7

Understanding Potassium 7

    What is Potassium? 7

    Role of Potassium in the Body 8

    Why a Potassium Diet? 9

Chapter Three: 10

Medical Aspects of Potassium in Seniors 10

    Common Health Conditions Requiring a Low Potassium Diet 10

        Chronic Kidney Disease (CKD) 10

        Heart Conditions 11

        Diabetes and Potassium Management 11

        Practical Dietary Management 12

    The Impact of High Potassium Levels 13

        Understanding Hyperkalemia 13

        Symptoms and Dangers of High Potassium Levels 13

        Causes of Hyperkalemia in Seniors 14

        Diagnosing Hyperkalemia 14

        Managing and Treating High Potassium Levels 14

        The Importance of Awareness and Education 15

    Consulting Healthcare Providers 15

    The Importance of Team-Based Healthcare 16

    Role of Primary Care Physicians 16

    Specialist Consultations 16

    The Role of Dietitians 17

    Importance of Pharmacists 17

    Regular Monitoring and Adjustments 17

    Communicating Effectively with Healthcare Providers 18

    Empowering Patients Through Education 18

Chapter Four: 19

The Basics of a Low Potassium Diet 19

    What Foods to Avoid 19

        Understanding Potassium in Foods 19

        High-Potassium Foods to Avoid 19

    Understanding Food Labels 22

        Serving Size and Servings per Container 22

        Understanding Micronutrients 23

        Tips for Navigating Food Labels 24

    Supplements and Senior Health 25

        Understanding Supplement Needs in Seniors 25

        Factors Influencing Nutrient Absorption 26

        Benefits of Supplements for Seniors 26

        Considerations for Supplement Use 27

Chapter Five: 29

Food List and Shopping Guide 29

    Detailed Low Potassium Food List 29

    Seasonal Food Guide 30

Benefits of Seasonal Eating: 31

Strategies for Seasonal Eating: 32

Breakfast 34

Greek Yogurt Parfait 34

Spinach and Feta Omelette 35

Banana Nut Overnight Oats 36

Vegetable Frittata 36

Whole Grain Pancakes 37

Mango Coconut Chia Pudding 38

Sweet Potato Breakfast Hash 39

Blueberry Almond Smoothie 40

Egg Muffins with Spinach and Feta 41

Apple Cinnamon Quinoa Breakfast Bowl 42

Lunch Recipes 44

Quinoa Salad with Chickpeas and Lemon Tahini Dressing 44

Vegetable Stir-Fry with Tofu 45

Mediterranean Chickpea Salad 46

Turkey and Avocado Wrap 47

Salmon and Quinoa Bowl 48

Black Bean and Corn Salad 49

Chicken Caesar Salad 50

Veggie and Hummus Wrap 51

Caprese Salad with Balsamic Glaze 52

Tuna Salad Stuffed with Bell Peppers 53

Dinner Recipes 55

Grilled Salmon with Roasted Vegetables 55

Vegetable Stir-Fried Noodles 56

Baked Chicken Parmesan 57

Vegetarian Chili with Quinoa 58

Lemon Garlic Shrimp Pasta 59

Vegetable and Tofu Stir-Fry 60

Roast Chicken with Sweet Potatoes and Brussels Sprouts 61

Beef and Broccoli Stir-Fry 62

Pesto Pasta with Cherry Tomatoes 64

Cauliflower Steak with Herb Sauce 65

Snacks 67

Cucumber and Hummus Plate 67

Apple and Peanut Butter Slices 67

Carrot Sticks with Ranch Dip 68

Cherry Tomato and Mozzarella Skewers 69

Greek Yogurt with Berries 70

Celery Sticks with Almond Butter 71

Cheese and Crackers 71

Air-popped popcorn with Olive Oil Spray 72

Roasted Chickpeas 73

Zucchini Chips 74

Beverages 75

Cucumber Mint Water 75

Lemon Basil Iced Tea 76

Cranberry Spritzer 76

Apple Cider Vinegar Tonic 77

Herbal Berry Infusion 78

Coconut Water with Lime 79

Peppermint Iced Tea 80

Ginger Lemonade 81

Strawberry Basil Sparkler 82

Blueberry Vanilla Smoothie 82

Homemade Crackers 84

Rosemary Olive Oil Crackers 84

Whole Wheat Sesame Crackers 85

Garlic Parmesan Crackers 86

Cheddar Chive Crackers 87

Spelt and Poppy Seed Crackers 88

Multi-Grain Crackers 89

Pumpkin Seed and Oat Crackers 90

Herb and Garlic Fiber Crackers 91

Caraway Rye Crackers 92

Cornmeal Lime Crackers 93

Smoothies 94

Berry Blast Smoothie 94

Green Goddess Smoothie 94

Tropical Paradise Smoothie 95

Banana Oat Smoothie 96

Creamy Peach Smoothie 97

Carrot Cake Smoothie 97

Chocolate Banana Protein Smoothie 98

Coconut Berry Smoothie 99

Vanilla Almond Smoothie 100

    Minty Watermelon Smoothie 101

Chapter Six: 102

30 Days Meal Plan 102

Chapter Seven:...113

Managing Diet Over Time 113

    Understanding the Need for Dietary Adjustments: 113

    Practical Tips for Adjusting the Diet:.. 114

    Long-term Monitoring of Potassium Levels 115

        Understanding Potassium Balance: 116

        Factors Affecting Potassium Levels: 116

        The Importance of Long-Term Monitoring:............................... 117

        Monitoring Methods: 117

        Interpreting Potassium Levels: 118

        Clinical Implications and Interventions:..................................... 118

        Long-Term Management Strategies: 119

Chapter Eight: 120

Conclusion 120

INTRODUCTION

Making wise decisions that improve one's quality of life is a key component of comprehending and putting into practice a low-potassium diet. Controlling dietary potassium is important, especially for older adults, but it's still one of the less-talked-about parts of maintaining senior health. The purpose of this introduction is to explain the fundamentals of a low-potassium diet, its significance, and how it can play a key role in maintaining general health in old age.

Potassium is a mineral that, under normal circumstances, plays a vital role in keeping the body healthy. It aids in the function of nerves and muscles, including the heart. Every heartbeat is regulated, in part, by potassium, which orchestrates the rhythmic contractions and relaxations. Additionally, potassium helps to balance fluids in the body and manages the movement of nutrients and waste into and out of cells, a fundamental process for cellular function.

However, while potassium is indispensable, its levels need to be carefully regulated, particularly in seniors. The ability of the body to handle potassium efficiently can diminish with age due to reduced kidney function or other underlying health conditions such as hypertension, diabetes, or heart issues. When kidneys are unable to efficiently remove excess potassium from the blood, the risk of hyperkalemia—where potassium levels become too high—increases, potentially leading to serious health consequences. These may include muscle weakness, confusion, heart palpitations, and in severe cases, life-threatening cardiac irregularities.

Thus, a low-potassium diet becomes essential for those whose bodies cannot regulate this mineral effectively. This diet involves careful consideration of food choices to avoid excessive potassium intake. It sounds simple but requires a nuanced understanding of nutrition and the potassium content of foods.

Most people know that bananas are rich in potassium, but there are less obvious sources like avocados, nuts, seeds, and certain vegetables such as spinach and broccoli. Furthermore, many processed foods contain added potassium, making label reading an essential skill for managing a low-potassium diet.

A low-potassium diet can be difficult to follow at first. But with the correct information and resources, it may become enjoyable to try new foods and flavors in addition to being manageable. This book aims to demystify the process and provide practical advice, from identifying low-potassium foods to understanding food labels and managing meals outside the home. The goal is not merely to adhere to a list of dietary restrictions but to embrace a healthy, satisfying diet that supports long-term well-being.

The challenge often lies not in the 'avoidance' but in balancing a diet that still meets all nutritional needs. Seniors, in particular, require diets that support bone health, manage blood pressure, and maintain muscle mass and cognitive function. It's about creating meals that are as nourishing as they are delicious, providing joy and variety at the dining table. This book will serve as a companion in that journey. It will offer detailed lists of foods tailored for a low-potassium regimen, practical shopping guides, and seasonal food suggestions to keep meals exciting and varied. More than that, it will provide a collection of recipes designed to make every meal a delight—from invigorating breakfasts to nutritious, hearty dinners.

Each recipe and guideline has been crafted with the understanding that diet is profoundly personal and evolves with our health needs. For seniors adjusting to a low-potassium diet, the transformation in eating habits can be significant but incredibly rewarding. The emphasis here is on ease and education, ensuring that each reader can confidently navigate their dietary needs without stress or confusion.

Finally, managing a diet over time is crucial, especially as health needs change. This book will discuss how to monitor potassium levels and adjust diets as necessary in consultation with healthcare providers. The aim is not only to provide a foundation for a low-potassium diet but also to ensure that it can be a sustainable, enjoyable part of a senior's lifestyle. Adopting a low-potassium diet is about improving life quality, one meal at a time, not just about going by a list of food dos and don'ts. Cooking is a true fusion of science and art, and with the correct knowledge and a little imagination, it can open up a new world of gastronomic delights while protecting health.

CHAPTER ONE:
IMPORTANCE OF POTASSIUM REGULATION IN SENIORS

Regulating potassium intake is crucial at any age, but for seniors, it holds particular significance due to the pivotal role it plays in overall health and the potential complications associated with its mismanagement. The delicate balance of potassium is not merely a dietary concern but a cornerstone of physiological wellness, especially as the body ages.

Potassium, a vital mineral and electrolyte in the human body, is essential for maintaining a range of biological functions. It helps to regulate the heartbeat, ensures proper function of the muscles and nerves, and is crucial for digesting carbohydrates and building protein. The balance of potassium powers the electrical charges that maintain heart rhythm and nerve function.

However, as we age, the body's ability to process potassium can become compromised due to diminished kidney function—the primary regulator of potassium. Aging kidneys filter blood less effectively, which can lead to either an accumulation or a rapid depletion of potassium. Both extremes pose significant health risks and managing these levels becomes increasingly important for elderly individuals.

Hyperkalemia: The Risks of High Potassium

Hyperkalemia, or high blood potassium, is a common issue faced by the elderly. It can occur due to the kidneys' reduced ability to excrete potassium, the effects of medications like ACE inhibitors or beta-blockers, or due to a diet high in potassium-rich foods. The symptoms of hyperkalemia include muscle weakness, fatigue, and heart palpitations. More severe cases can lead to dangerous heart arrhythmias and even sudden cardiac arrest.

Seniors are particularly susceptible to these risks, not only because of natural changes in kidney function but also because of the prevalence of chronic diseases that affect renal health and the likelihood of multiple medication use. Thus, monitoring and regulating potassium intake becomes a critical aspect of managing older adults' health.

Hypokalemia: The Dangers of Low Potassium

Conversely, hypokalemia, or low blood potassium, can also be particularly dangerous for seniors. It may result from conditions such as excessive fluid loss through prolonged vomiting, diarrhea, or the use of diuretics. Symptoms of hypokalemia include muscle cramps, weakness, fatigue, and constipation. Severe hypokalemia can impair muscle function and heart health, leading to arrhythmias and even cardiac arrest.

The Role of Diet and Medication

Managing potassium levels in seniors is not merely about adjusting dietary intake. It also involves careful monitoring of medications that impact potassium levels. Diuretics, commonly prescribed for hypertension in seniors, can significantly lower potassium levels, while certain blood pressure medications can increase them. Regular blood tests are crucial to ensure potassium levels are kept within a safe range, and dietary adjustments may be required based on these results.

Dietary Management: A Preventive Approach

For many seniors, dietary management is a first line of defense in preventing potassium imbalances. This includes education about potassium-rich foods, such as bananas, oranges, potatoes, and spinach, and guidance on alternatives that maintain nutritional balance without exacerbating health issues. It is about making informed choices that consider both the nutritional content and the specific health needs of the individual.

Nutritionists and dietitians play a crucial role in crafting eating plans that address these concerns while ensuring that the diet remains enjoyable and varied. Seniors and their caregivers need to understand not only what foods to limit but also how to create satisfying meals that promote health. This dietary strategy not only prevents disease but also enhances the quality of life by promoting an optimal balance of nutrients.

Education and Empowerment

Empowering seniors with knowledge about how their bodies change with age and how to adapt their diets can significantly improve their quality of life and independence. Educational programs and resources that focus on dietary management, the importance of regular medical checkups, and the impact of medications on potassium levels are essential. These programs help demystify medical terminology and make the science of nutrition more accessible.

CHAPTER TWO:
UNDERSTANDING POTASSIUM

What is Potassium?

Potassium is a vital mineral that plays numerous crucial roles in the human body. It is classified as an electrolyte because it is highly reactive in water and produces positively charged ions. This characteristic enables it to conduct electricity, which is essential for many bodily functions, particularly in the cells of muscle tissue and the nervous system.

Potassium is found naturally in many foods and is also available as a dietary supplement. The human body requires potassium to maintain normal cell function, and it is one of the key electrolytes that help regulate heartbeat and muscle function, including the smooth muscles and muscles involved in breathing.

In addition to its role in muscle function and nerve transmission, potassium is crucial for maintaining fluid balance within the cells and throughout the body. It works in concert with sodium to maintain normal blood pressure and is also involved in protein synthesis and carbohydrate metabolism, which are crucial for overall health and energy levels.

Because the body does not produce potassium naturally, it must be obtained through diet. The kidneys play a key role in managing blood potassium levels, removing excess amounts through urine. Thus, maintaining a balance of potassium is essential as both excessive and inadequate potassium levels can lead to serious health issues.

Role of Potassium in the Body

The significance of potassium in the body is vast and multifaceted. One of the primary roles of potassium is in maintaining cellular function through the regulation of fluid balance. This is done in balance with sodium and chloride to ensure that cells neither shrink nor swell, an imbalance that can lead to cellular and organ dysfunction.

On a larger scale, potassium is crucial for cardiovascular health. It helps to regulate heart rate and ensures proper electrical signaling in the heart, which prevents irregular heartbeats, known as arrhythmias. Studies have shown that adequate potassium intake can reduce the risk of stroke by lowering blood pressure and counteracting the adverse effects of sodium.

Moreover, potassium aids in nutrient metabolism, helping with the conversion of glucose into glycogen which can be stored in the liver for energy. It is also vital for muscle health, not just for the contractions of skeletal muscle but also for smooth muscle found in organs like the digestive tract, where it helps to facilitate digestion and regulate bowel movements.

In the nervous system, potassium is essential for the propagation of nerve signals, known as action potentials. These are the signals that control everything from reflexes to complex maneuvers, as well as the proper functioning of the brain. Adequate potassium levels are thus essential for cognitive functions such as memory and learning.

Why a Potassium Diet?

A low-potassium diet is often prescribed for individuals who cannot rid their bodies of excess potassium efficiently, a common issue among those with kidney disease. When the kidneys are compromised, they may not filter potassium properly from the blood, leading to hyperkalemia, a condition where potassium levels in the blood are higher than normal, which can be dangerous.

Symptoms of hyperkalemia can be mild at lower levels, such as numbness or weakness, and life-threatening at higher levels, including heart palpitations or cardiac arrest. For patients with chronic kidney disease or conditions that affect potassium excretion, managing dietary potassium intake becomes crucial to avoid these risks.

Furthermore, certain medications commonly prescribed for heart disease, like ACE inhibitors and potassium-sparing diuretics, can increase potassium levels in the blood. In such cases, a low potassium diet helps to keep potassium levels within a safe range, complementing the medication regimen and mitigating potential adverse effects.

Adjusting one's diet to lower potassium intake requires careful planning to ensure nutritional balance is maintained. Foods that are typically high in potassium include bananas, oranges, potatoes, spinach, and tomatoes. Choices, such as apples, berries, carrots, and lettuce, are lower in potassium and safer for individuals requiring restricted intake.

CHAPTER THREE:
MEDICAL ASPECTS OF POTASSIUM IN SENIORS

As individuals age, the management of potassium becomes increasingly important due to the critical roles this essential mineral plays in the human body. Potassium helps regulate heart function, muscle contractions, and nerve signals. But, in seniors, the stakes are higher as their bodies face challenges in maintaining the delicate balance required for optimal health. This is particularly pertinent when considering common health conditions that necessitate a low-potassium diet.

Common Health Conditions Requiring a Low Potassium Diet

In the elderly, several prevalent health conditions make potassium management a priority. Chronic kidney disease (CKD), heart conditions, and diabetes are among the most common ailments that may require adjustments in dietary potassium. Understanding these conditions and their interaction with potassium can help tailor dietary strategies to better support senior health.

Chronic Kidney Disease (CKD)
Chronic kidney disease is one of the leading health concerns in seniors that necessitates a careful watch over potassium intake. As kidney function declines with age or disease, the ability of these organs to filter

out excess potassium diminishes. This can lead to hyperkalemia, where potassium levels in the blood become dangerously high, potentially leading to cardiac arrest or other serious health issues.

In managing CKD, a low-potassium diet is often prescribed to help prevent the accumulation of potassium to harmful levels. Seniors with CKD must monitor their potassium intake rigorously, avoiding high-potassium foods and being mindful of hidden potassium in processed foods. The diet should be carefully balanced to ensure that while potassium is limited, other nutritional needs are met to maintain overall health.

Heart Conditions

Potassium plays a significant role in heart health by helping to regulate heartbeat and muscle function. However, in cases of heart disease, particularly those involving heart failure or conditions treated with certain types of heart medications such as ACE inhibitors or beta-blockers, potassium levels need to be carefully managed.

These medications can increase potassium retention, which, while beneficial in some aspects, can pose risks if potassium levels become too high. For seniors with these conditions, a low potassium diet may be necessary to keep potassium at a safe level and prevent complications like arrhythmias—a disorder of the heart rate or rhythm.

Diabetes and Potassium Management

Potassium level complications can also result from diabetes, a frequent ailment among the elderly. Potassium is transported from the bloodstream into cells by insulin, and variations in insulin levels—which are prevalent in diabetes—can cause problems with potassium homeostasis. Furthermore, the risk of hyperkalemia is raised by the renal damage that frequently results from high blood sugar levels associated with diabetes, which further complicates potassium excretion.

For diabetic seniors, managing carbohydrate intake and maintaining blood sugar levels is crucial, but so is monitoring and managing potassium intake. Ensuring that dietary potassium does not reach excessive levels while also caring for their diabetic condition requires careful planning and continuous monitoring.

Practical Dietary Management

Managing these conditions involves not just understanding the diseases themselves but also how they interact with dietary elements like potassium. For nutritionists and healthcare providers, crafting a diet low in potassium for seniors with these health concerns involves detailed knowledge of both the nutritional content of food and the specific health needs of the individual.

Education plays a vital role in managing health through diet. Seniors and their caregivers need practical knowledge about which foods are high in potassium and which are safer choices. This education also extends to understanding food labels, recognizing the symptoms of both hyperkalemia and hypokalemia and knowing when to seek medical advice.

Furthermore, regular monitoring of potassium levels through blood tests is essential for seniors with health conditions affecting potassium balance. This allows for timely adjustments to the diet or medication to ensure potassium levels remain within a safe range.

The Impact of High Potassium Levels

Potassium, a critical electrolyte in the human body, plays vital roles in a variety of physiological processes, including the regulation of heartbeat, muscle function, and nerve transmission. While maintaining adequate levels of potassium is essential for health, an excess of this mineral can lead to significant health issues, especially in vulnerable populations such as seniors. High potassium levels, or hyperkalemia, can have far-reaching effects on the body, necessitating both an understanding of the risks involved and strategies to mitigate them.

Understanding Hyperkalemia

Hyperkalemia occurs when potassium in the bloodstream exceeds normal levels. For most adults, the normal range for potassium is between 3.5 and 5.0 millimoles per liter (mmol/L). Levels above 5.5 mmol/L are generally considered to be hyperkalemic and can pose serious health risks. The body usually maintains potassium levels within a tight range through the kidneys, which filter excess potassium out of the blood and excrete it in urine. However, certain conditions, particularly those affecting kidney function, can impair this process, leading to the accumulation of potassium.

Symptoms and Dangers of High Potassium Levels

The symptoms of hyperkalemia can vary and often depend on the level of potassium in the blood. Mildly elevated levels may not produce any symptoms at all, making regular monitoring important for those at risk. As levels increase, symptoms can become more pronounced and may include muscle weakness, fatigue, and tingling sensations. One of the most dangerous aspects of hyperkalemia is its effect on the heart. High potassium levels can alter the normal electrical activity of the heart, leading to irregular heartbeats, which can be fatal if not treated promptly.

Causes of Hyperkalemia in Seniors

In seniors, the most common cause of hyperkalemia is impaired kidney function. With age, kidney function naturally declines, and the organs become less efficient at filtering potassium from the blood. Chronic kidney disease (CKD), which is prevalent among older adults, exacerbates this problem. Other factors contributing to hyperkalemia in seniors include medications that affect kidney function or potassium levels, such as ACE inhibitors, angiotensin receptor blockers, and certain diuretics used to treat high blood pressure and heart conditions.

Diagnosing Hyperkalemia

Diagnosing hyperkalemia involves blood tests to measure potassium levels. Given the potential for hyperkalemia to be asymptomatic, especially in its early stages, regular blood tests are critical for those at risk. Electrocardiograms (ECG) may also be used to detect changes in heart rhythm that can indicate severe hyperkalemia.

Managing and Treating High Potassium Levels

The management of hyperkalemia focuses on both acute and long-term strategies. In acute cases, where potassium levels are dangerously high, prompt medical treatment is necessary to prevent cardiac complications.

Treatments may include medications that stabilize heart rhythms, intravenous calcium to counteract the effects of potassium on the heart, and agents that shift potassium from the blood into cells.

For long-term management, dietary adjustments are essential. Patients are advised to avoid foods high in potassium, such as bananas, oranges, potatoes, and spinach. Education on reading food labels and recognizing potassium additives in processed foods is also crucial.

Besides dietary management, medications may require adjustment. For those whose hyperkalemia is linked to medications, doctors may reduce dosages or switch to alternative treatments that have a lesser impact on potassium levels. Regular monitoring through blood tests remains a cornerstone of managing hyperkalemia, ensuring that any adjustments to diet or medication maintain potassium levels within a safe range.

The Importance of Awareness and Education

Education about hyperkalemia and its potential impacts is vital, not only for those at risk but also for caregivers and family members. Understanding the signs of elevated potassium levels, knowing when to seek medical help, and how to manage diet and medication can significantly reduce the risks associated with hyperkalemia.

Consulting Healthcare Providers

In managing the health of older adults, particularly when it comes to balancing essential nutrients like potassium, the role of healthcare providers is indispensable. Potassium, vital for many cellular functions, needs careful monitoring in seniors due to their susceptibility to both hyperkalemia (high potassium levels) and hypokalemia (low potassium levels). Consulting with healthcare providers—ranging from general practitioners to specialists in cardiology, nephrology, and dietetics—is crucial for maintaining optimal potassium levels and ensuring overall well-being.

The Importance of Team-Based Healthcare

Managing potassium levels in seniors often requires a team-based approach. This team may include primary care physicians, kidney specialists (nephrologists), heart specialists (cardiologists), pharmacists, and registered dietitians. Each professional brings a different perspective and expertise, providing a comprehensive approach to potassium management. The primary care physician often coordinates this care, ensuring that all aspects of the senior's health are considered and that treatments from different specialists do not conflict.

Role of Primary Care Physicians

The primary care physician is typically the first point of contact for seniors experiencing health issues. They play a pivotal role in the initial assessment and monitoring of potassium levels, especially in patients who are at risk due to conditions like chronic kidney disease, cardiovascular disease, or diabetes. These physicians are responsible for conducting initial blood tests, prescribing and managing basic treatments, and referring patients to specialists when needed.

Specialist Consultations

For more complex cases, such as those where kidney function or heart health is severely compromised, specialists are integral. Nephrologists help manage kidney health and are crucial in adjusting treatments that impact kidney function and potassium excretion. Cardiologists are essential for managing the risks that fluctuating potassium levels pose to heart health, especially in patients with a history of heart disease.

The Role of Dietitians

Dietitians specialize in nutrition and provide essential guidance on how dietary choices affect potassium levels. They work closely with patients to create personalized eating plans that manage potassium intake, which is vital for patients diagnosed with hyperkalemia or at risk of it. Dietitians also educate patients and their families about which foods are high in potassium, how to read and understand food labels, and strategies to maintain a balanced diet while managing potassium levels.

Importance of Pharmacists

Pharmacists also play a crucial role, particularly in understanding the complex interactions between medications and potassium levels. Many seniors take multiple medications, and pharmacists are pivotal in ensuring that these do not adversely affect potassium levels. They can provide advice on the timing of medication doses to minimize the impact on potassium and suggest alternatives if current prescriptions are affecting potassium balance.

Regular Monitoring and Adjustments

Consulting healthcare providers is not a one-time activity but a continuous process. Regular follow-ups and monitoring are essential, especially for seniors with conditions that affect potassium levels. These check-ups allow healthcare providers to track the effectiveness of treatments and make necessary adjustments. Blood tests are a routine part of these follow-ups, helping to ensure that potassium levels remain within a safe range and adjusting treatment plans as the patient's health status changes.

Communicating Effectively with Healthcare Providers

Effective communication is crucial in managing health care, especially for seniors managing potassium levels. Patients and their caregivers need to be open and honest about their dietary habits, medication adherence, and any symptoms they might be experiencing. This transparency allows healthcare providers to offer the most effective care.

Additionally, seniors and their families should be prepared to ask questions and express concerns during consultations. Understanding the reasons behind certain dietary restrictions, medication prescriptions, or treatments can enhance adherence to prescribed health regimens and lead to better health outcomes.

Empowering Patients Through Education

Healthcare providers also have a role in educating patients about the importance of potassium management. By providing patients with information about why maintaining potassium levels is critical and how it can be achieved, healthcare providers empower patients to take an active role in their health management.

CHAPTER FOUR:

THE BASICS OF A LOW POTASSIUM DIET

What Foods to Avoid

For seniors and individuals managing certain health conditions, such as kidney disease or heart issues, adhering to a low-potassium diet is often a critical component of their health regimen. Potassium, an essential mineral, plays a vital role in many bodily functions, including nerve function and muscle contraction. However, when potassium levels become too high, due to reduced kidney function or other factors, it can lead to serious health complications, including heart arrhythmias and muscle weakness. Understanding which foods to avoid is key to managing and maintaining healthy potassium levels.

Understanding Potassium in Foods

Potassium is naturally present in many foods, especially fruits, vegetables, whole grains, and meats. While these foods are generally considered healthy, they can pose risks for individuals who need to manage their potassium intake. The first step in adhering to a low-potassium diet is identifying high-potassium foods to limit or avoid.

High-Potassium Foods to Avoid

1. **Fruits**

Certain fruits are particularly high in potassium and should be consumed sparingly or avoided by those on a low-potassium diet:

- **Bananas:** One of the most well-known high-potassium foods, bananas should be avoided.

- **Oranges and Orange Juice:** Both the fruit and its juice are high in potassium.

- **Avocados:** Very rich in potassium, avocados are typically restricted on a low-potassium diet.

- **Dried fruits:** Such as apricots, prunes, and raisins, are concentrated sources of potassium.

2. Vegetables

Some vegetables also contain high levels of potassium and should be limited:

- **Potatoes and Sweet Potatoes:** Both contain high potassium levels, though leaching (soaking cut potatoes in water) can reduce their potassium content.

- **Tomatoes:** Including raw tomatoes, tomato sauce, and tomato juice.

- **Spinach and Swiss Chard:** These leafy greens are high in potassium, especially when cooked, as they concentrate their mineral content.

- **Beet Greens and Beets:** Known for their high potassium levels.

3. Legumes and Nuts

These are nutritious but also high in potassium:

- **Beans:** Including kidney beans, pinto beans, and black beans.

- **Lentils:** While healthy, they are typically high in potassium and should be avoided on a strict low-potassium diet.
- **Nuts and Seeds:** Particularly almonds, pistachios, and sunflower seeds are high in potassium.

4. Dairy Products

Dairy products can vary in potassium content, but generally:

- **Milk and Yogurt:** Both are high in potassium, and intake should be monitored or alternatives sought.
- **Cheese:** Some cheeses are also high in potassium, though portion control can help manage intake.

5. Meat and Fish

While meat and fish are essential sources of protein, some are high in potassium:

- **Red Meat:** Generally higher in potassium than chicken or turkey.
- **Certain Fish:** Such as salmon, cod, and halibut, have higher potassium levels.

6. Whole Grains

Whole grains are generally healthier than refined grains but can have higher potassium levels:

- **Whole Wheat Products and Bran Cereals:** These can be higher in potassium compared to their more processed counterparts.

Understanding Food Labels

Food labels are an essential tool for individuals striving to make informed dietary choices, especially those on specialized diets like a low potassium regimen. While they may seem complex at first glance, understanding how to decipher food labels is a valuable skill that empowers individuals to manage their nutritional intake effectively. This comprehensive guide aims to demystify food labels, providing insight into the key components and considerations for those navigating a low-potassium diet.

Serving Size and Servings per Container

The serving size listed on the food label represents the amount typically consumed in one sitting. It is crucial to compare this serving size to the amount you consume to accurately assess the nutritional content. Additionally, the number of servings per container informs how many servings are contained within the entire package.

Calories

Calories indicate the amount of energy provided by the food. While calorie intake is important for overall health, it is equally vital to consider the source of those calories and their nutritional value.

Macronutrients: Fat, Carbohydrates, and Protein

Fat, carbohydrates, and protein are macronutrients that provide essential nutrients and energy. Understanding the breakdown of these macronutrients can help individuals make informed dietary choices. For example, opting for foods lower in saturated and trans fats can promote heart health, while choosing complex carbohydrates over simple sugars can help maintain stable blood sugar levels.

Dietary Fiber

Dietary fiber is an important component of a healthy diet, aiding in digestion and promoting bowel regularity. Foods high in fiber, such as fruits, vegetables, and whole grains, are often beneficial for individuals managing a low-potassium diet.

Sugars

Monitoring sugar intake is crucial, especially for individuals with conditions like diabetes or those aiming to reduce calorie consumption. Pay attention to both natural sugars, found in fruits and dairy products, and added sugars, which may contribute to excess calorie intake without providing nutritional benefits.

Understanding Micronutrients

Sodium

Sodium intake is closely linked to potassium levels, making it particularly relevant for individuals on a low-potassium diet. High sodium intake can exacerbate potassium retention in the body, leading to elevated potassium levels. Monitoring sodium content in processed foods and choosing low-sodium alternatives can help maintain a healthy balance.

Potassium

While potassium is not always listed on food labels, certain ingredients may indicate higher potassium content. Ingredients such as potassium chloride, potassium bicarbonate, or potassium citrate are indicators of added potassium and should be monitored by individuals managing potassium intake.

Vitamins and Minerals

Food labels often provide information on the vitamins and minerals present in the product. Pay attention to micronutrients like calcium, magnesium, and vitamin D, which are important for bone health and overall well-being. While not directly related to potassium management, ensuring adequate intake of these nutrients contributes to overall health.

Tips for Navigating Food Labels

Read Ingredients Lists

In addition to the nutritional facts panel, examining the ingredients list can provide valuable insight into the composition of the food product. Ingredients are listed in descending order by weight, with the primary ingredient listed first. Be wary of additives or preservatives that may contribute to potassium content.

Use Reference Materials

Utilize resources such as dietary guidelines, nutrition databases, or smartphone apps to gather information on the nutritional content of specific foods. These tools can help identify low-potassium alternatives and support informed decision-making.

Be Mindful of Portion Sizes

Even low-potassium foods can contribute to elevated potassium levels if consumed in large quantities. Pay attention to portion sizes and consider how they fit into your overall dietary plan.

Choose Whole, Minimally Processed Foods

Whole foods, such as fruits, vegetables, lean proteins, and whole grains, are often naturally lower in potassium and provide essential nutrients without added preservatives or additives.

Supplements and Senior Health

As individuals age, their nutritional needs may change due to factors such as decreased appetite, changes in metabolism, and reduced absorption of nutrients. While a balanced diet rich in whole foods is the foundation of good health, supplements can play a valuable role in addressing specific nutritional deficiencies and supporting overall well-being in seniors. This comprehensive exploration delves into the benefits, considerations, and recommendations for supplement use in senior health.

Understanding Supplement Needs in Seniors

Seniors are more prone to certain nutritional deficiencies, including:

- **Vitamin D:** Reduced sun exposure and decreased skin synthesis of vitamin D contribute to deficiencies, impacting bone health and immune function.

- **Calcium:** Inadequate intake of calcium can lead to bone loss and increase the risk of osteoporosis.

- **Vitamin B12:** Decreased stomach acid production and gastrointestinal changes can impair absorption of vitamin B12, impacting nerve function and red blood cell production.
- **Omega-3 Fatty Acids:** Low intake of fatty fish and other sources of omega-3s can affect cognitive function and cardiovascular health.

Factors Influencing Nutrient Absorption

Various factors can affect nutrient absorption in seniors, including:

- **Gastrointestinal Changes:** Aging can lead to changes in stomach acid production, digestive enzyme activity, and intestinal absorption, impacting nutrient uptake.
- **Medication Interactions:** Certain medications may interfere with nutrient absorption or increase nutrient excretion, necessitating higher intake or supplementation.
- **Dental Health:** Poor dental health or missing teeth can affect chewing and digestion, reducing nutrient absorption from food.

Benefits of Supplements for Seniors

Supplements can help bridge the gap between dietary intake and nutrient requirements, ensuring seniors receive adequate levels of essential vitamins and minerals. This is particularly important for individuals with restricted diets or those with difficulty chewing or swallowing, which may limit food choices.

Supporting Bone Health

Calcium and vitamin D supplements are crucial for maintaining bone density and reducing the risk of fractures in seniors, especially those with osteoporosis or at risk of falls. Adequate calcium and vitamin D intake support bone formation and calcium absorption, promoting skeletal health and preventing fractures.

Enhancing Cognitive Function

Omega-3 fatty acids, particularly docosahexaenoic acid (DHA) and eicosapentaenoic acid (EPA) have been linked to cognitive health and may help reduce the risk of cognitive decline and dementia in seniors. Omega-3 supplements derived from fish oil or algae can support brain function and memory, contributing to overall cognitive well-being.

Supporting Immune Function

Vitamins and minerals like vitamin C, vitamin E, zinc, and selenium play essential roles in immune function and may help bolster the body's defenses against infections and illness. Supplementation with these nutrients can support immune health in seniors, particularly during periods of increased susceptibility, such as cold and flu season.

Considerations for Supplement Use

Supplement needs vary among seniors based on factors such as age, gender, health status, and medication use. A personalized approach, guided by healthcare providers, ensures that supplements are tailored to individual needs and goals.

Quality and Safety

Choosing high-quality supplements from reputable manufacturers is paramount to ensure efficacy and safety. Look for products that have been tested by third-party organizations for purity, potency, and quality assurance.

Potential Interactions

Seniors should be mindful of potential interactions between supplements and medications they may be taking. Certain supplements, such as vitamin K, can interfere with blood-thinning medications like warfarin, while others may enhance or diminish the effects of prescription drugs.

Dosage and Timing

Optimal dosing and timing of supplements can vary based on individual needs and health conditions. Healthcare providers can offer guidance on the appropriate dosage, timing, and frequency of supplement intake to maximize benefits and minimize risks.

CHAPTER FIVE:
FOOD LIST AND SHOPPING GUIDE

Detailed Low Potassium Food List

Food Group	Low Potassium Foods
Fruits	Apples, Berries (e.g., strawberries, blueberries), Grapes, Pineapple, Peaches, Pears, Cherries, Mangoes, Papayas, Watermelon (in moderation)
Vegetables	Bell Peppers, Cabbage, Carrots, Cauliflower, Cucumber, Eggplant, Lettuce, Onions (in moderation), Peas (green), Zucchini
Grains	White Bread (enriched), White Rice, Pasta (refined), Cornflakes, Oats (moderate consumption), Barley (in moderation)
Protein Sources	Eggs, Chicken (skinless, white meat), Turkey (skinless, white meat), Beef (lean cuts, in moderation), Pork (lean cuts, in moderation), Tofu, Tempeh, Seitan, Lentils, White Beans
Dairy and Alternatives	Milk (non-dairy, fortified with calcium and low in potassium), Yogurt (low-fat or non-fat), Cheese (low-fat varieties and in moderation), Almond Milk

	(unsweetened), Rice Milk, Coconut Milk (unsweetened)
Snacks and Sweets	Popcorn (plain, air-popped), Pretzels (unsalted), Rice Cakes, Graham Crackers, Vanilla Wafers, Sorbet (fruit-flavored, low potassium), Gelatin (unflavored), Hard Candy (in moderation)
Beverages	Water, Herbal Tea (caffeine-free), Lemonade (made with low potassium fruits), Apple Juice (diluted and in moderation), Cranberry Juice (unsweetened and in moderation)
Fats and Oils	Olive Oil, Canola Oil, Margarine (low-sodium and low-potassium varieties), Butter (in moderation)
Condiments and Seasonings	Salt (in moderation), Pepper, Herbs (fresh or dried), Spices (e.g., garlic powder, onion powder, paprika), Vinegar (white, apple cider)
Miscellaneous	Jams and Jellies (low potassium varieties), Honey (in moderation), Maple Syrup (pure), Pickles (low-sodium and in moderation), Mustard (prepared, low-sodium)

Seasonal Food Guide

Taking advantage of the abundant harvest of each season is not only a healthy but also an environmentally responsible way to choose food when it comes to mindful eating and sustainable eating. A seasonal food guide directs customers toward locally sourced produce that is at its freshest and tastiest. It functions like a compass. Let's explore how using a seasonal food guide might enhance your culinary explorations and what advantages it offers.

Benefits of Seasonal Eating:

1. **Optimal Nutrition:** Seasonal produce is typically harvested at its peak ripeness, maximizing its nutritional content. Fresh fruits and vegetables are rich in essential vitamins, minerals, and antioxidants, promoting overall health and well-being.

2. **Enhanced Flavor:** Fruits and vegetables allowed to ripen naturally and picked at the peak of freshness boast superior flavor profiles. From juicy summer berries to crisp autumn apples, seasonal eating tantalizes the taste buds with vibrant, natural flavors.

3. **Environmental Sustainability:** Embracing seasonal eating reduces the carbon footprint associated with food production and transportation. By supporting local farmers and consuming locally grown produce, individuals contribute to a more sustainable food system.

4. **Cost-Effectiveness:** In-season produce is often more abundant and therefore more affordable than out-of-season varieties. Shopping for seasonal ingredients can help stretch your food budget without compromising on quality or flavor.

Strategies for Seasonal Eating:

1. **Consult a Seasonal Food Guide:** Stay informed about what fruits and vegetables are in season in your region by referring to seasonal food guides available online, in cookbooks, or from local agricultural extension offices. These guides highlight the peak seasons for various crops, helping you plan your meals accordingly.

2. **Shop at Farmers' Markets:** Farmers' markets are treasure troves of seasonal produce, offering a diverse array of fruits, vegetables, and herbs directly from local growers. Engage with farmers to learn about their growing practices and discover new seasonal favorites.

3. **Join a Community Supported Agriculture (CSA) Program:** CSA programs provide subscribers with weekly or monthly deliveries of seasonal produce directly from local farms. By participating in a CSA, you not only enjoy a variety of fresh, seasonal produce but also support small-scale agriculture in your community.

4. **Preserve the Harvest:** Extend the enjoyment of seasonal produce by preserving excess fruits and vegetables through methods such as canning, freezing, or drying. Homemade jams, pickles, and frozen berries allow you to savor the flavors of summer long after the season has passed.

5. **Experiment with Seasonal Recipes:** Embrace the creativity of seasonal cooking by exploring new recipes that highlight the

flavors of in-season produce. From refreshing salads and hearty soups to decadent desserts, seasonal ingredients can inspire culinary delights for every palate.

BREAKFAST

Greek Yogurt Parfait

Prep Time: 5 minutes

Cooking Time: 0 minutes

Serving Size: 1

Ingredients:

- 1/2 cup Greek yogurt (plain, low-fat)
- 1/4 cup granola (low-sugar)
- 1/2 cup mixed berries (strawberries, blueberries, raspberries)
- 1 tablespoon honey (optional)

Instructions:

1. In a serving glass or bowl, layer Greek yogurt, granola, and mixed berries.
2. Drizzle with honey if desired.

Nutritional Information (per serving):

- Calories: 250
- Protein: 15g
- Sodium: 80mg
- Potassium: 300mg
- Phosphorus: 200mg

Spinach and Feta Omelette

Prep Time: 5 minutes

Cooking Time: 5 minutes

Serving Size: 1

Ingredients:

- 2 eggs
- 1/2 cup fresh spinach (chopped)
- 2 tablespoons crumbled feta cheese
- Pinch of black pepper
- Pinch of garlic powder

Instructions:

1. In a bowl, whisk together eggs, spinach, and feta cheese.
2. Heat a non-stick skillet over medium heat and pour in the egg mixture.
3. Cook until the edges start to set, then fold the omelet in half.
4. Cook for another 1-2 minutes until the cheese is melted and the eggs are cooked through.

Nutritional Information (per serving):

- Calories: 280
- Protein: 20g
- Sodium: 300mg
- Potassium: 250mg
- Phosphorus: 300mg

Banana Nut Overnight Oats

Prep Time: 5 minutes

Cooking Time: 0 minutes

Serving Size: 1

Ingredients:
- 1/2 cup rolled oats
- 1/2 cup almond milk (unsweetened)
- 1/2 ripe banana (mashed)
- 1 tablespoon chopped nuts (walnuts, almonds)
- 1 teaspoon honey or maple syrup (optional)

Instructions:
1. In a jar or bowl, combine rolled oats, almond milk, mashed banana, and chopped nuts.
2. Stir well to combine, then cover and refrigerate overnight.
3. In the morning, stir the oats and add honey or maple syrup if desired.

Nutritional Information (per serving):
- Calories: 320
- Protein: 9g
- Sodium: 80mg
- Potassium: 350mg

Vegetable Frittata

Prep Time: 10 minutes

Cooking Time: 15 minutes

Serving Size: 1

Ingredients:

- 2 eggs
- 1/4 cup diced bell peppers (red, yellow, green)
- 1/4 cup diced tomatoes
- 2 tablespoons diced onions
- 1 tablespoon chopped fresh herbs (parsley, basil)
- Pinch of salt and black pepper

Instructions:

1. Preheat the oven to 350°F (175°C).
2. In a bowl, whisk together eggs, diced vegetables, chopped herbs, salt, and pepper.
3. Pour the egg mixture into a greased oven-safe skillet.
4. Bake for 12-15 minutes until the frittata is set and the edges are golden brown.
5. Slice and serve warm.

Nutritional Information (per serving):

- Calories: 200
- Protein: 12g
- Sodium: 220mg
- Potassium: 250mg
- Phosphorus: 200mg

Whole Grain Pancakes

Prep Time: 10 minutes

Cooking Time: 10 minutes

Serving Size: 1

Ingredients:

- 1/2 cup whole wheat flour
- 1/2 teaspoon baking powder
- 1/4 teaspoon cinnamon
- 1/2 cup almond milk (unsweetened)
- 1 tablespoon maple syrup

Instructions:

1. In a bowl, whisk together whole wheat flour, baking powder, and cinnamon.
2. Stir in almond milk and maple syrup until smooth.
3. Heat a non-stick skillet over medium heat and lightly grease with cooking spray.
4. Pour batter onto the skillet to form pancakes.
5. Cook for 2-3 minutes on each side until golden brown.
6. Serve with fresh fruit or yogurt if desired.

Nutritional Information (per serving):

- Calories: 220
- Protein: 6g
- Sodium: 180mg
- Potassium: 150mg
- Phosphorus: 100mg

Mango Coconut Chia Pudding

Prep Time: 5 minutes

Cooking Time: 0 minutes

Serving Size: 1

Ingredients:

- 1/4 cup chia seeds
- 1/2 cup coconut milk (unsweetened)
- 1/2 cup diced mango
- 1 tablespoon shredded coconut (unsweetened)
- 1 teaspoon vanilla extract

Instructions:

1. In a jar or bowl, combine chia seeds, coconut milk, diced mango, shredded coconut, and vanilla extract.
2. Stir well to combine, then cover and refrigerate for at least 2 hours or overnight.
3. Stir the pudding before serving and top with additional mango or coconut if desired.

Nutritional Information (per serving):

- Calories: 280
- Protein: 6g
- Sodium: 20mg
- Potassium: 200mg
- Phosphorus: 150mg

Sweet Potato Breakfast Hash

Prep Time: 10 minutes

Cooking Time: 20 minutes

Serving Size: 1

Ingredients:

- 1 small sweet potato (diced)
- 1/4 cup diced bell peppers (any color)
- 1/4 cup diced onions
- 1/4 cup black beans (canned, rinsed and drained)
- 1/4 teaspoon smoked paprika
- Pinch of salt and black pepper

Instructions:

1. Heat a skillet over medium heat and add diced sweet potato.
2. Cook for 5-7 minutes until the sweet potato starts to soften.
3. Add diced bell peppers, onions, black beans, smoked paprika, salt, and pepper to the skillet.
4. Cook for another 8-10 minutes until the vegetables are tender and lightly browned.
5. Serve hot with a side of scrambled eggs or avocado slices if desired.

Nutritional Information (per serving):

- Calories: 240
- Protein: 7g
- Sodium: 200mg
- Potassium: 350mg

Blueberry Almond Smoothie

Prep Time: 5 minutes

Cooking Time: 0 minutes

Serving Size: 1

Ingredients:

- 1/2 cup frozen blueberries
- 1/2 banana (frozen for creaminess)
- 1/4 cup Greek yogurt (plain, low-fat)
- 1 tablespoon almond butter
- 1/2 cup almond milk (unsweetened)
- 1 teaspoon honey or maple syrup (optional)

Instructions:

1. In a blender, combine frozen blueberries, bananas, Greek yogurt, almond butter, almond milk, and honey or maple syrup if desired.
2. Blend until smooth and creamy.
3. Pour into a glass and enjoy immediately.

Nutritional Information (per serving):

- Calories: 280
- Protein: 9g
- Sodium: 80mg
- Potassium: 350mg
- Phosphorus: 200mg

Egg Muffins with Spinach and Feta

Prep Time: 10 minutes

Cooking Time: 20 minutes

Serving Size: 1

Ingredients:
- 2 eggs
- 1/4 cup chopped spinach (fresh or frozen)
- 2 tablespoons crumbled feta cheese
- Pinch of black pepper
- Pinch of garlic powder

Instructions:
1. Preheat the oven to 350°F (175°C) and grease a muffin tin.
2. In a bowl, whisk together eggs, chopped spinach, feta cheese, black pepper, and garlic powder.
3. Pour the egg mixture into the prepared muffin tin, filling each cup about 2/3 full.
4. Bake for 15-20 minutes until the egg muffins are set and lightly golden.
5. Allow to cool slightly before serving.

Nutritional Information (per serving):
- Calories: 180
- Protein: 12g
- Sodium: 250mg
- Potassium: 200mg
- Phosphorus: 150mg

Apple Cinnamon Quinoa Breakfast Bowl

Prep Time: 5 minutes
Cooking Time: 15 minutes

Serving Size: 1

Ingredients:

- 1/2 cup cooked quinoa
- 1/2 apple (diced)
- 2 tablespoons chopped walnuts
- 1/2 teaspoon cinnamon
- 1 tablespoon maple syrup or honey
- 1/4 cup almond milk (unsweetened)

Instructions:

1. In a bowl, combine cooked quinoa, diced apple, chopped walnuts, cinnamon, maple syrup or honey, and almond milk.
2. Stir well to combine.
3. Microwave for 1-2 minutes until heated through.
4. Serve hot and enjoy.

Nutritional Information (per serving):

- Calories: 300
- Protein: 8g
- Sodium: 80mg
- Potassium: 250mg
- Phosphorus: 150mg

LUNCH RECIPES

Quinoa Salad with Chickpeas and Lemon Tahini Dressing

Prep Time: 10 minutes

Cooking Time: 15 minutes

Serving Size: 1

Ingredients:

- 1/2 cup cooked quinoa
- 1/2 cup canned chickpeas (rinsed and drained)
- 1/4 cup diced cucumber
- 1/4 cup diced tomatoes
- 2 tablespoons chopped fresh parsley
- 2 tablespoons lemon tahini dressing

Instructions:

1. In a bowl, combine cooked quinoa, chickpeas, cucumber, tomatoes, and parsley.
2. Drizzle with lemon tahini dressing and toss to coat evenly.

Nutritional Information (per serving):

- Calories: 350
- Protein: 12g
- Sodium: 200mg

- Potassium: 350mg
- Phosphorus: 250mg

Vegetable Stir-Fry with Tofu

Prep Time: 10 minutes

Cooking Time: 15 minutes

Serving Size: 1

Ingredients:

- 1/2 cup diced tofu
- 1/2 cup mixed vegetables (bell peppers, broccoli, snap peas)
- 2 tablespoons low-sodium soy sauce
- 1 tablespoon sesame oil
- 1 teaspoon minced garlic
- 1/2 teaspoon grated ginger

Instructions:

1. Heat sesame oil in a skillet over medium heat.
2. Add minced garlic and grated ginger, and sauté for 1 minute.
3. Add diced tofu and cook until golden brown.
4. Add mixed vegetables and soy sauce, and stir-fry until vegetables are tender-crisp.

Nutritional Information (per serving):

- Calories: 280
- Protein: 15g

- Sodium: 400mg
- Potassium: 350mg
- Phosphorus: 200mg

Mediterranean Chickpea Salad

Prep Time: 10 minutes

Cooking Time: 0 minutes

Serving Size: 1

Ingredients:

- 1/2 cup canned chickpeas (rinsed and drained)
- 1/4 cup diced cucumber
- 1/4 cup diced tomatoes
- 2 tablespoons diced red onion
- 2 tablespoons chopped fresh parsley
- 1 tablespoon olive oil
- 1 tablespoon lemon juice
- Pinch of salt and black pepper

Instructions:

1. In a bowl, combine chickpeas, cucumber, tomatoes, red onion, and parsley.
2. Drizzle with olive oil and lemon juice, and season with salt and black pepper. Toss to combine.

Nutritional Information (per serving):

- Calories: 250

- Protein: 9g
- Sodium: 300mg
- Potassium: 350mg
- Phosphorus: 150mg

Turkey and Avocado Wrap

Prep Time: 10 minutes

Cooking Time: 0 minutes

Serving Size: 1

Ingredients:

- 2 slices whole grain wrap or tortilla
- 2 ounces sliced turkey breast
- 1/4 avocado (sliced)
- 1/4 cup shredded lettuce
- 2 slices tomato
- 1 tablespoon hummus

Instructions:

1. Lay out the whole grain wrap or tortilla.
2. Layer sliced turkey breast, avocado, shredded lettuce, tomato, and hummus.
3. Roll up tightly and slice in half if desired.

Nutritional Information (per serving):

- Calories: 300

- Protein: 20g
- Sodium: 400mg
- Potassium: 350mg
- Phosphorus: 200mg

Salmon and Quinoa Bowl

Prep Time: 10 minutes

Cooking Time: 15 minutes

Serving Size: 1

Ingredients:

- 1/2 cup cooked quinoa
- 4 ounces grilled or baked salmon fillet
- 1/2 cup steamed broccoli florets
- 1/4 cup shredded carrots
- 1 tablespoon soy sauce
- 1 teaspoon sesame seeds

Instructions:

1. In a bowl, layer cooked quinoa, grilled salmon, steamed broccoli, and shredded carrots.
2. Drizzle with soy sauce and sprinkle with sesame seeds.

Nutritional Information (per serving):

- Calories: 350
- Protein: 25g

- Sodium: 400mg
- Potassium: 450mg
- Phosphorus: 250mg

Black Bean and Corn Salad

Prep Time: 10 minutes

Cooking Time: 0 minutes

Serving Size: 1

Ingredients:

- 1/2 cup canned black beans (rinsed and drained)
- 1/4 cup corn kernels (fresh or frozen)
- 2 tablespoons diced red bell pepper
- 2 tablespoons diced green bell pepper
- 2 tablespoons chopped fresh cilantro
- 1 tablespoon lime juice
- 1 tablespoon olive oil
- Pinch of salt and cumin

Instructions:

1. In a bowl, combine black beans, corn kernels, diced bell peppers, and chopped cilantro.
2. Drizzle with lime juice and olive oil, and season with salt and cumin. Toss to combine.

Nutritional Information (per serving):

- Calories: 220

- Protein: 8g
- Sodium: 200mg
- Potassium: 300mg
- Phosphorus: 150mg

Chicken Caesar Salad

Prep Time: 10 minutes

Cooking Time: 15 minutes

Serving Size: 1

Ingredients:

- 2 cups chopped romaine lettuce
- 4 ounces grilled chicken breast (sliced)
- 2 tablespoons grated Parmesan cheese
- 2 tablespoons Caesar dressing (low-fat)
- 1/4 cup croutons (whole grain)

Instructions:

- In a large bowl, toss together chopped romaine lettuce, sliced grilled chicken breast, grated Parmesan cheese, and Caesar dressing.
- Top with whole-grain croutons before serving.

Nutritional Information (per serving):

- Calories: 280
- Protein: 30g

- Sodium: 400mg
- Potassium: 350mg
- Phosphorus: 250mg

Veggie and Hummus Wrap

Prep Time: 10 minutes

Cooking Time: 0 minutes

Serving Size: 1

Ingredients:

- 2 slices whole grain wrap or tortilla
- 2 tablespoons hummus
- 1/4 cup shredded carrots
- 1/4 cup sliced cucumber
- 1/4 cup sliced bell peppers
- 1/4 cup baby spinach leaves

Instructions:

1. Lay out the whole grain wrap or tortilla.
2. Spread hummus evenly over the wrap.
3. Layer shredded carrots, sliced cucumber, sliced bell peppers, and baby spinach leaves.
4. Roll up tightly and slice in half if desired.

Nutritional Information (per serving):

- Calories: 250

- Protein: 8g
- Sodium: 300mg
- Potassium: 350mg
- Phosphorus: 200mg

Caprese Salad with Balsamic Glaze

Prep Time: 10 minutes

Cooking Time: 0 minutes

Serving Size: 1

Ingredients:

- 1/2 cup cherry tomatoes (halved)
- 1/4 cup fresh mozzarella balls (bocconcini)
- 2 tablespoons fresh basil leaves (torn)
- 1 tablespoon balsamic glaze
- Pinch of salt and black pepper

Instructions:

1. In a bowl, combine cherry tomatoes, fresh mozzarella balls, and torn basil leaves.
2. Drizzle with balsamic glaze and season with salt and black pepper. Toss to combine.

Nutritional Information (per serving):

- Calories: 220
- Protein: 10g

- Sodium: 300mg
- Potassium: 350mg
- Phosphorus: 200mg

Tuna Salad Stuffed with Bell Peppers

Prep Time: 10 minutes

Cooking Time: 0 minutes

Serving Size: 1

Ingredients:

- 1 bell pepper (halved and seeds removed)
- 1/2 cup canned tuna (drained)
- 2 tablespoons diced celery
- 2 tablespoons diced red onion
- 1 tablespoon plain Greek yogurt
- 1 teaspoon Dijon mustard
- Pinch of salt and black pepper

Instructions:

1. In a bowl, combine canned tuna, diced celery, diced red onion, Greek yogurt, Dijon mustard, salt, and black pepper.
2. Spoon the tuna salad mixture into the halved bell pepper.
3. Serve immediately or refrigerate until ready to eat.

Nutritional Information (per serving):

- Calories: 200

- Protein: 25g
- Sodium: 350mg
- Potassium: 400mg
- Phosphorus: 250mg

DINNER RECIPES

Grilled Salmon with Roasted Vegetables

Prep Time: 10 minutes
Cooking Time: 20 minutes
Serving Size: 1

Ingredients:

- 4 ounces salmon fillet
- 1 cup mixed vegetables (bell peppers, zucchini, cherry tomatoes)
- 1 tablespoon olive oil
- 1 teaspoon dried herbs (rosemary, thyme)
- Pinch of salt and black pepper

Instructions:

1. Preheat the grill to medium-high heat.
2. Brush salmon fillet and mixed vegetables with olive oil.
3. Season with dried herbs, salt, and black pepper.
4. Grill salmon for 4-5 minutes on each side until cooked through.
5. Roast mixed vegetables in the oven at 400°F (200°C) for 15-20 minutes.

Nutritional Information (per serving):

- Calories: 350
- Protein: 25g
- Sodium: 300mg

- Potassium: 450mg
- Phosphorus: 250mg

Vegetable Stir-Fried Noodles

Prep Time: 10 minutes

Cooking Time: 15 minutes

Serving Size: 1

Ingredients:

- 2 ounces whole wheat noodles (cooked)
- 1 cup mixed vegetables (broccoli, carrots, snap peas)
- 2 tablespoons low-sodium soy sauce
- 1 tablespoon sesame oil
- 1 teaspoon minced garlic
- 1/2 teaspoon grated ginger

Instructions:

1. Heat sesame oil in a wok or skillet over medium heat.
2. Add minced garlic and grated ginger, and stir-fry for 1 minute.
3. Add mixed vegetables and cook until tender-crisp.
4. Toss in cooked noodles and soy sauce, and stir-fry until well combined.

Nutritional Information (per serving):

- Calories: 300
- Protein: 10g
- Sodium: 400mg

- Potassium: 350mg
- Phosphorus: 200mg

Baked Chicken Parmesan

Prep Time: 15 minutes

Cooking Time: 25 minutes

Serving Size: 1

Ingredients:

- 4 ounces chicken breast (boneless, skinless)
- 1/4 cup whole wheat breadcrumbs
- 2 tablespoons grated Parmesan cheese
- 1/4 cup marinara sauce (low-sodium)
- 1/4 cup shredded mozzarella cheese (part-skim)
- 1 tablespoon chopped fresh basil

Instructions:

1. Preheat the oven to 400°F (200°C).
2. In a shallow dish, combine whole wheat breadcrumbs and grated Parmesan cheese.
3. Coat chicken breast in breadcrumb mixture, then place on a baking sheet.
4. Bake for 20 minutes, then top with marinara sauce and shredded mozzarella cheese.
5. Bake for an additional 5 minutes until cheese is melted and bubbly.

Nutritional Information (per serving):

- Calories: 350
- Protein: 30g
- Sodium: 400mg
- Potassium: 350mg
- Phosphorus: 250mg

Vegetarian Chili with Quinoa

Prep Time: 15 minutes

Cooking Time: 30 minutes

Serving Size: 1

Ingredients:

- 1/4 cup uncooked quinoa
- 1 cup canned black beans (rinsed and drained)
- 1 cup canned kidney beans (rinsed and drained)
- 1 cup diced tomatoes (canned or fresh)
- 1/2 cup diced bell peppers
- 1/2 cup diced onions
- 2 cloves garlic (minced)
- 1 tablespoon chili powder
- 1 teaspoon cumin
- Pinch of salt and black pepper

Instructions:

1. Cook quinoa according to package instructions.
2. In a large pot, sauté diced onions and bell peppers until softened.
3. Add minced garlic, chili powder, cumin, salt, and black pepper, and cook for 1 minute.
4. Stir in diced tomatoes, black beans, kidney beans, and cooked quinoa.
5. Simmer for 20-25 minutes until flavors are combined and chili is thickened.

Nutritional Information (per serving):

- Calories: 300
- Protein: 15g
- Sodium: 400mg
- Potassium: 450mg
- Phosphorus: 200mg

Lemon Garlic Shrimp Pasta

Prep Time: 10 minutes

Cooking Time: 15 minutes

Serving Size: 1

Ingredients:

- 2 ounces whole wheat spaghetti (cooked)
- 4 ounces shrimp (peeled and deveined)
- 1 tablespoon olive oil

- 2 cloves garlic (minced)
- 1 tablespoon lemon juice
- 1/4 teaspoon red pepper flakes
- Pinch of salt and black pepper

Instructions:

1. Cook whole wheat spaghetti according to package instructions.
2. In a skillet, heat olive oil over medium heat.
3. Add minced garlic and red pepper flakes, and sauté for 1 minute.
4. Add shrimp to the skillet and cook until pink and cooked through.
5. Stir in cooked spaghetti and lemon juice, and season with salt and black pepper.

Nutritional Information (per serving):

- Calories: 320
- Protein: 20g
- Sodium: 400mg
- Potassium: 350mg
- Phosphorus: 200mg

Vegetable and Tofu Stir-Fry

Prep Time: 10 minutes
Cooking Time: 15 minutes
Serving Size: 1

Ingredients:

- 2 ounces tofu (extra firm, diced)

- 1 cup mixed vegetables (bell peppers, broccoli, carrots)
- 2 tablespoons low-sodium soy sauce
- 1 tablespoon hoisin sauce
- 1 teaspoon sesame oil
- 1 teaspoon cornstarch (dissolved in 1 tablespoon water)

Instructions:
1. Heat sesame oil in a wok or skillet over medium heat.
2. Add diced tofu and cook until golden brown on all sides.
3. Add mixed vegetables and stir-fry until tender.
4. Combine low-sodium soy sauce, hoisin sauce, and cornstarch mixture.
5. Add to the wok and stir until the sauce thickens and coats the vegetables and tofu.

Nutritional Information (per serving):
- Calories: 280
- Protein: 12g
- Sodium: 400mg
- Potassium: 350mg
- Phosphorus: 250mg

Roast Chicken with Sweet Potatoes and Brussels Sprouts

Prep Time: 10 minutes
Cooking Time: 35 minutes
Serving Size: 1
Ingredients:

- 4 ounces chicken thigh (boneless, skinless)

- 1/2 cup sweet potatoes (cubed)
- 1/2 cup Brussels sprouts (halved)
- 1 tablespoon olive oil
- 1 teaspoon paprika
- Pinch of salt and black pepper

Instructions:

1. Preheat the oven to 375°F (190°C).
2. Toss the sweet potatoes and Brussels sprouts in olive oil, paprika, salt, and black pepper.
3. Place the vegetables on one half of a baking sheet.
4. On the other half, place the chicken thigh, seasoning it similarly with olive oil, paprika, salt, and black pepper.
5. Roast in the oven for 35 minutes, or until the chicken is cooked through and the vegetables are tender and caramelized.

Nutritional Information (per serving):

- Calories: 350
- Protein: 22g
- Sodium: 300mg
- Potassium: 400mg
- Phosphorus: 200mg

Beef and Broccoli Stir-Fry

Prep Time: 10 minutes

Cooking Time: 15 minutes

Serving Size: 1

Ingredients:

- 4 ounces beef (sirloin, thinly sliced)
- 1 cup broccoli florets
- 1 tablespoon soy sauce (low sodium)
- 1 teaspoon sesame oil
- 1 clove garlic (minced)
- 1/2 teaspoon grated ginger
- 1 teaspoon cornstarch (dissolved in 2 tablespoons water)

Instructions:

1. Heat sesame oil in a wok or skillet over medium-high heat.
2. Add minced garlic and grated ginger, stir-frying briefly until fragrant.
3. Add the beef and cook until it starts to brown.
4. Add broccoli and continue to stir-fry until vegetables are tender.
5. Mix soy sauce and cornstarch water in a small bowl, then pour over the beef and broccoli.
6. Stir until the sauce has thickened and everything is well coated.

Nutritional Information (per serving):

- Calories: 350
- Protein: 25g
- Sodium: 400mg
- Potassium: 400mg
- Phosphorus: 250mg

Pesto Pasta with Cherry Tomatoes

Prep Time: 5 minutes

Cooking Time: 10 minutes

Serving Size: 1

Ingredients:

- 2 ounces whole wheat spaghetti
- 1/4 cup homemade or store-bought pesto (low sodium)
- 1/2 cup cherry tomatoes (halved)
- 1 tablespoon grated Parmesan cheese

Instructions:

1. Cook spaghetti according to package directions.
2. Drain pasta and return to pot.
3. Stir in pesto and cherry tomatoes until well combined and heated through.
4. Serve topped with grated Parmesan cheese.

Nutritional Information (per serving):

- Calories: 320
- Protein: 10g
- Sodium: 200mg
- Potassium: 300mg
- Phosphorus: 150mg

Cauliflower Steak with Herb Sauce

Prep Time: 10 minutes

Cooking Time: 25 minutes

Serving Size: 1

Ingredients:

- 1 large cauliflower slice (1-inch thick)
- 2 tablespoons olive oil
- 1/4 cup fresh herbs (parsley, cilantro, dill)
- 1 clove garlic (minced)
- 1 tablespoon lemon juice
- Pinch of salt and black pepper

Instructions:

1. Preheat the oven to 400°F (200°C).
2. Brush both sides of the cauliflower steak with olive oil and season with salt and pepper.
3. Roast in the preheated oven for about 25 minutes, flipping halfway through, until golden and tender.
4. Blend fresh herbs, minced garlic, lemon juice, and a bit more olive oil to create a sauce.
5. Serve the roasted cauliflower topped with the fresh herb sauce.

Nutritional Information (per serving):

- Calories: 250
- Protein: 5g

- Sodium: 200mg
- Potassium: 500mg
- Phosphorus: 150mg

SNACKS

Cucumber and Hummus Plate

Prep Time: 5 minutes

Cooking Time: 0 minutes

Serving Size: 1

Ingredients:

- 1 medium cucumber, sliced
- 1/4 cup hummus
- Instructions:
- Slice the cucumber.
- Serve with a side of hummus for dipping.

Nutritional Information (per serving):

- Calories: 180
- Protein: 6g
- Sodium: 260mg
- Potassium: 250mg
- Phosphorus: 120mg

Apple and Peanut Butter Slices

Prep Time: 5 minutes

Cooking Time: 0 minutes

Serving Size: 1

Ingredients:

- 1 medium apple, cored and sliced
- 1 tablespoon peanut butter

Instructions:

1. Core and slice the apple.
2. Spread peanut butter on each slice.

Nutritional Information (per serving):

- Calories: 200
- Protein: 4g
- Sodium: 70mg
- Potassium: 200mg
- Phosphorus: 100mg

Carrot Sticks with Ranch Dip

Prep Time: 5 minutes

Cooking Time: 0 minutes

Serving Size: 1

Ingredients:

- 1 cup carrot sticks
- 1/4 cup low-sodium ranch dressing

Instructions:

1. Cut carrots into sticks.
2. Serve with ranch dressing for dipping.

Nutritional Information (per serving):

- Calories: 150
- Protein: 2g
- Sodium: 320mg
- Potassium: 320mg
- Phosphorus: 50mg

Cherry Tomato and Mozzarella Skewers

Prep Time: 10 minutes

Cooking Time: 0 minutes

Serving Size: 1

Ingredients:

- 5 cherry tomatoes
- 5 small mozzarella balls
- Fresh basil leaves
- Balsamic glaze (optional)

Instructions:

1. Skewer alternating cherry tomatoes, mozzarella balls, and basil leaves on small sticks.
2. Drizzle with balsamic glaze if desired.

Nutritional Information (per serving):

- Calories: 200
- Protein: 8g
- Sodium: 180mg
- Potassium: 150mg
- Phosphorus: 90mg

Greek Yogurt with Berries

Prep Time: 5 minutes

Cooking Time: 0 minutes

Serving Size: 1

Ingredients:

- 1/2 cup plain Greek yogurt
- 1/4 cup mixed berries (blueberries, raspberries)

Instructions:

1. Spoon yogurt into a bowl.
2. Top with mixed berries.

Nutritional Information (per serving):

- Calories: 150
- Protein: 12g
- Sodium: 45mg
- Potassium: 200mg
- Phosphorus: 150mg

Celery Sticks with Almond Butter

Prep Time: 5 minutes

Cooking Time: 0 minutes

Serving Size: 1

Ingredients:

- 3 celery stalks, trimmed
- 1 tablespoon almond butter

Instructions:

1. Trim celery stalks and clean them.
2. Spread almond butter inside the celery grooves.

Nutritional Information (per serving):

- Calories: 100
- Protein: 3g
- Sodium: 80mg
- Potassium: 300mg
- Phosphorus: 100mg

Cheese and Crackers

Prep Time: 5 minutes

Cooking Time: 0 minutes

Serving Size: 1

Ingredients:

- 4 whole-grain crackers
- 2 slices of low-sodium cheese

Instructions:

1. Place cheese slices on crackers.

Nutritional Information (per serving):

- Calories: 150
- Protein: 6g
- Sodium: 200mg
- Potassium: 100mg
- Phosphorus: 120mg

Air-popped popcorn with Olive Oil Spray

Prep Time: 2 minutes

Cooking Time: 3 minutes

Serving Size: 1

Ingredients:

- 1/3 cup popcorn kernels
- Olive oil spray
- Pinch of salt

Instructions:

2. Pop the kernels using an air popper.

3. Lightly spray with olive oil and sprinkle with a pinch of salt.

Nutritional Information (per serving):

- Calories: 100
- Protein: 3g
- Sodium: 50mg
- Potassium: 75mg
- Phosphorus: 90mg

Roasted Chickpeas

Prep Time: 5 minutes

Cooking Time: 20 minutes

Serving Size: 1

Ingredients:

- 1/2 cup chickpeas, drained and rinsed
- 1 teaspoon olive oil
- 1/2 teaspoon smoked paprika

Instructions:

1. Preheat oven to 400°F (200°C).
2. Toss chickpeas with olive oil and smoked paprika.
3. Spread on a baking sheet and roast for 20 minutes until crispy.

Nutritional Information (per serving):

- Calories: 150
- Protein: 6g

- Sodium: 200mg
- Potassium: 210mg
- Phosphorus: 120mg

Zucchini Chips

Prep Time: 10 minutes

Cooking Time: 20 minutes

Serving Size: 1

Ingredients:

- 1 small zucchini, thinly sliced
- 1 teaspoon olive oil
- Pinch of salt

Instructions:

1. Preheat oven to 400°F (200°C).
2. Toss zucchini slices in olive oil and a pinch of salt.
3. Arrange in a single layer on a baking sheet.
4. Bake for 20 minutes, flipping halfway through until crispy.

Nutritional Information (per serving):

- Calories: 60
- Protein: 2g
- Sodium: 50mg
- Potassium: 290mg
- Phosphorus: 50mg

BEVERAGES

Cucumber Mint Water

Prep Time: 5 minutes

Cooking Time: 0 minutes

Serving Size: 1

Ingredients:

- 1/2 cucumber, thinly sliced
- 5 mint leaves
- 1 liter of water

Instructions:

1. Add cucumber slices and mint leaves to a pitcher of water.
2. Chill for at least an hour before serving to enhance the flavors.

Nutritional Information (per serving):

- Calories: 0
- Protein: 0g
- Sodium: 10mg
- Potassium: 40mg
- Phosphorus: 0mg

Lemon Basil Iced Tea

Prep Time: 5 minutes

Cooking Time: 5 minutes

Serving Size: 1

Ingredients:

- 1 tea bag (black or green tea)
- 1/4 lemon, sliced
- 3 fresh basil leaves
- 1 cup boiling water

Instructions:

1. Steep the tea bag, lemon slices, and basil leaves in boiling water for 5 minutes.
2. Remove the tea bag and let it cool. Serve over ice.

Nutritional Information (per serving):

- Calories: 2
- Protein: 0g
- Sodium: 0mg
- Potassium: 30mg
- Phosphorus: 0mg

Cranberry Spritzer

Prep Time: 5 minutes

Cooking Time: 0 minutes

Serving Size: 1

Ingredients:

- 1/2 cup cranberry juice (low sugar)
- 1/2 cup sparkling water
- Ice cubes
- Lime wedge, for garnish

Instructions:

1. Mix cranberry juice with sparkling water.
2. Serve over ice and garnish with a lime wedge.

Nutritional Information (per serving):

- Calories: 60
- Protein: 0g
- Sodium: 5mg
- Potassium: 30mg
- Phosphorus: 0mg

Apple Cider Vinegar Tonic

Prep Time: 5 minutes

Cooking Time: 0 minutes

Serving Size: 1

Ingredients:

- 1 tablespoon apple cider vinegar
- 1 teaspoon honey
- 1 cup water
- Ice cubes

Instructions:

1. Mix apple cider vinegar and honey in water until well combined.
2. Serve over ice.

Nutritional Information (per serving):

- Calories: 25
- Protein: 0g
- Sodium: 5mg
- Potassium: 30mg
- Phosphorus: 0mg

Herbal Berry Infusion

Prep Time: 5 minutes

Cooking Time: 10 minutes

Serving Size: 1

Ingredients:

- 1/4 cup mixed berries (blueberries, strawberries)
- 1 bag herbal tea (e.g., chamomile)
- 1 cup boiling water

Instructions:

1. Place berries and an herbal tea bag in a cup.
2. Pour boiling water over and steep for 10 minutes.
3. Strain and serve warm or chilled.

Nutritional Information (per serving):

- Calories: 30
- Protein: 0g
- Sodium: 0mg
- Potassium: 40mg
- Phosphorus: 0mg

Coconut Water with Lime

Prep Time: 5 minutes

Cooking Time: 0 minutes

Serving Size: 1

Ingredients:

- 1 cup coconut water
- Juice of 1/2 lime
- Ice cubes

Instructions:

1. Mix coconut water with lime juice.
2. Serve over ice.

Nutritional Information (per serving):

- Calories: 46
- Protein: 0g
- Sodium: 25mg
- Potassium: 60mg
- Phosphorus: 0mg

Peppermint Iced Tea

Prep Time: 5 minutes

Cooking Time: 10 minutes

Serving Size: 1

Ingredients:

- 1 peppermint tea bag
- 1 cup boiling water
- Ice cubes

Instructions:

1. Steep peppermint tea bag in boiling water for 10 minutes.
2. Remove the tea bag and let it cool. Serve over ice.

Nutritional Information (per serving):

- Calories: 0
- Protein: 0g
- Sodium: 0mg
- Potassium: 0mg

- Phosphorus: 0mg

Ginger Lemonade

Prep Time: 10 minutes

Cooking Time: 0 minutes

Serving Size: 1

Ingredients:

- 1 teaspoon grated ginger
- 1/2 lemon, juiced
- 1 teaspoon honey
- 1 cup water
- Ice cubes

Instructions:

1. Mix grated ginger, lemon juice, honey, and water.
2. Strain the mixture to remove the ginger fibers.
3. Serve over ice.

Nutritional Information (per serving):

- Calories: 20
- Protein: 0g
- Sodium: 0mg
- Potassium: 10mg
- Phosphorus: 0mg

Strawberry Basil Sparkler

Prep Time: 10 minutes

Cooking Time: 0 minutes

Serving Size: 1

Ingredients:

- 3 strawberries, sliced
- 2 basil leaves
- 1/2 cup sparkling water
- Ice cubes

Instructions:

1. Muddle strawberries and basil leaves in a glass.
2. Add ice cubes and top with sparkling water.

Nutritional Information (per serving):

- Calories: 15
- Protein: 0g
- Sodium: 0mg
- Potassium: 35mg
- Phosphorus: 0mg

Blueberry Vanilla Smoothie

Prep Time: 5 minutes

Cooking Time: 0 minutes

Serving Size: 1

- **Ingredients:**
- 1/4 cup blueberries
- 1/2 cup almond milk
- 1/2 teaspoon vanilla extract
- Ice cubes

Instructions:

1. Blend blueberries, almond milk, vanilla extract, and ice until smooth.

Nutritional Information (per serving):

- Calories: 50
- Protein: 1g
- Sodium: 30mg
- Potassium: 35mg
- Phosphorus: 20mg

HOMEMADE CRACKERS

Rosemary Olive Oil Crackers

Prep Time: 15 minutes

Cooking Time: 10 minutes

Serving Size: 10 crackers

Ingredients:

- 1 cup all-purpose flour
- 1/2 teaspoon salt
- 1 tablespoon fresh rosemary, finely chopped
- 3 tablespoons olive oil
- 1/4 cup water

Instructions:

- Preheat oven to 450°F (230°C).
- Combine flour, salt, and rosemary in a bowl.
- Add olive oil and water to form a dough.
- Roll out dough thinly and cut into desired shapes.
- Bake for 10 minutes or until golden and crisp.

Nutritional Information (per serving):

- Calories: 60
- Protein: 1g
- Sodium: 115mg

- Potassium: 20mg
- Phosphorus: 15mg

Whole Wheat Sesame Crackers

Prep Time: 15 minutes

Cooking Time: 15 minutes

Serving Size: 10 crackers

Ingredients:

- 1 cup whole wheat flour
- 1/4 teaspoon salt
- 2 tablespoons sesame seeds
- 3 tablespoons vegetable oil
- 1/3 cup water

Instructions:

2. Preheat oven to 350°F (175°C).
3. Mix flour, salt, and sesame seeds.
4. Stir in oil and water to form a stiff dough.
5. Roll out the dough and cut it into squares.
6. Bake for 15 minutes or until crisp.

Nutritional Information (per serving):

- Calories: 70
- Protein: 2g
- Sodium: 55mg

- Potassium: 40mg
- Phosphorus: 50mg

Garlic Parmesan Crackers

Prep Time: 15 minutes

Cooking Time: 12 minutes

Serving Size: 10 crackers

Ingredients:

- 1 cup all-purpose flour
- 1/2 teaspoon garlic powder
- 1/4 cup grated Parmesan cheese
- 4 tablespoons butter
- 2 tablespoons water

Instructions:

1. Preheat oven to 400°F (200°C).
2. Combine flour, garlic powder, and Parmesan in a bowl.
3. Cut in butter until the mixture resembles coarse crumbs.
4. Add water to form a dough.
5. Roll out thinly, cut into shapes, and bake for 12 minutes.

Nutritional Information (per serving):

- Calories: 80
- Protein: 2g
- Sodium: 75mg

- Potassium: 20mg
- Phosphorus: 30mg

Cheddar Chive Crackers

Prep Time: 10 minutes

Cooking Time: 15 minutes

Serving Size: 10 crackers

Ingredients:

- 1 cup all-purpose flour
- 1/2 cup shredded cheddar cheese
- 2 tablespoons chopped chives
- 4 tablespoons butter
- 3 tablespoons water

Instructions:

1. Preheat oven to 375°F (190°C).
2. Mix flour, cheese, and chives in a bowl.
3. Incorporate butter and then add water to form a dough.
4. Roll out and cut into desired shapes.
5. Bake for 15 minutes until crisp.

Nutritional Information (per serving):

- Calories: 85
- Protein: 3g
- Sodium: 95mg

- Potassium: 15mg
- Phosphorus: 40mg

Spelt and Poppy Seed Crackers

Prep Time: 15 minutes

Cooking Time: 10 minutes

Serving Size: 10 crackers

Ingredients:

- 1 cup spelt flour
- 1/2 teaspoon salt
- 1 tablespoon poppy seeds
- 3 tablespoons olive oil
- 1/4 cup water

Instructions:

1. Preheat oven to 425°F (220°C).
2. Combine spelt flour, salt, and poppy seeds.
3. Mix in olive oil and water to form a dough.
4. Roll out dough thinly, cut into shapes, and bake for 10 minutes.

Nutritional Information (per serving):

- Calories: 70
- Protein: 2g
- Sodium: 115mg
- Potassium: 30mg

- Phosphorus: 40mg

Multi-Grain Crackers

Prep Time: 20 minutes

Cooking Time: 18 minutes

Serving Size: 10 crackers

Ingredients:

- 1/2 cup whole wheat flour
- 1/4 cup oats
- 2 tablespoons flaxseeds
- 1/4 teaspoon salt
- 3 tablespoons vegetable oil
- 1/3 cup water

Instructions:

1. Preheat oven to 350°F (175°C).
2. Mix all dry ingredients.
3. Stir in oil and water to form a dough.
4. Roll out dough thinly, cut into shapes, and bake for 18 minutes.

Nutritional Information (per serving):

- Calories: 80
- Protein: 3g
- Sodium: 60mg
- Potassium: 50mg

- Phosphorus: 60mg

Pumpkin Seed and Oat Crackers

Prep Time: 15 minutes

Cooking Time: 15 minutes

Serving Size: 10 crackers

Ingredients:

- 1/2 cup rolled oats
- 1/4 cup pumpkin seeds
- 1/4 teaspoon salt
- 3 tablespoons sunflower oil
- 1/4 cup water

Instructions:

1. Preheat oven to 350°F (175°C).
2. Combine oats, pumpkin seeds, and salt in a food processor.
3. Add oil and water, pulsing to form a cohesive dough.
4. Roll out dough, cut into shapes, and bake for 15 minutes.

Nutritional Information (per serving):

- Calories: 80
- Protein: 3g
- Sodium: 50mg
- Potassium: 30mg
- Phosphorus: 70mg

Herb and Garlic Fiber Crackers

Prep Time: 15 minutes

Cooking Time: 12 minutes

Serving Size: 10 crackers

Ingredients:

- 1 cup fiber-rich flour blend
- 1/2 teaspoon garlic powder
- 1 tablespoon dried herbs (thyme, oregano)
- 4 tablespoons olive oil
- 1/4 cup water

Instructions:

1. Preheat oven to 400°F (200°C).
2. Mix flour, garlic powder, and herbs.
3. Add olive oil and water to form a dough.
4. Roll out thinly, cut into shapes, and bake for 12 minutes.

Nutritional Information (per serving):

- Calories: 70
- Protein: 2g
- Sodium: 50mg
- Potassium: 20mg
- Phosphorus: 30mg

Caraway Rye Crackers

Prep Time: 10 minutes

Cooking Time: 10 minutes

Serving Size: 10 crackers

Ingredients:

- 1 cup rye flour
- 1 teaspoon caraway seeds
- 1/4 teaspoon salt
- 3 tablespoons butter
- 2 tablespoons water

Instructions:

1. Preheat oven to 425°F (220°C).
2. Combine rye flour, caraway seeds, and salt.
3. Cut in butter until crumbly.
4. Add water to form a dough.
5. Roll out and cut into desired shapes. Bake for 10 minutes.

Nutritional Information (per serving):

- Calories: 70
- Protein: 2g
- Sodium: 55mg
- Potassium: 40mg
- Phosphorus: 50mg

Cornmeal Lime Crackers

Prep Time: 15 minutes

Cooking Time: 12 minutes

Serving Size: 10 crackers

Ingredients:

- 1 cup cornmeal
- 1/4 teaspoon salt
- Zest one lime
- 4 tablespoons vegetable oil
- 1/4 cup water

Instructions:

1. Preheat oven to 400°F (200°C).
2. Mix cornmeal, salt, and lime zest.
3. Stir in oil and water to form a dough.
4. Roll out thinly and cut into shapes.
5. Bake for 12 minutes until crisp.

Nutritional Information (per serving):

- Calories: 80
- Protein: 1g
- Sodium: 55mg
- Potassium: 25mg
- Phosphorus: 40mg

SMOOTHIES

Berry Blast Smoothie

Prep Time: 5 minutes

Serving Size: 1

Ingredients:

- 1/2 cup mixed berries (strawberries, blueberries, raspberries)
- 1/2 cup unsweetened almond milk
- 1/4 cup Greek yogurt (low-fat)
- 1 tablespoon honey (optional)

Instructions:

1. Combine all ingredients in a blender.
2. Blend until smooth.

Nutritional Information (per serving):

- Calories: 100
- Protein: 5g
- Sodium: 80mg
- Potassium: 150mg
- Phosphorus: 100mg

Green Goddess Smoothie

Prep Time: 5 minutes

Serving Size: 1

Ingredients:

- 1/2 ripe banana
- 1 cup spinach
- 1/2 cup unsweetened coconut milk
- 1 tablespoon almond butter

Instructions:

1. Blend all ingredients until smooth.

Nutritional Information (per serving):

- Calories: 150
- Protein: 4g
- Sodium: 120mg
- Potassium: 280mg
- Phosphorus: 80mg

Tropical Paradise Smoothie

Prep Time: 5 minutes

Serving Size: 1

Ingredients:

- 1/2 cup pineapple chunks
- 1/2 cup mango chunks
- 1/2 cup unsweetened coconut water
- 1/4 cup Greek yogurt (low-fat)

Instructions:

1. Blend all ingredients until smooth.

Nutritional Information (per serving):

- Calories: 120
- Protein: 3g
- Sodium: 30mg
- Potassium: 280mg
- Phosphorus: 80mg

Banana Oat Smoothie

Prep Time: 5 minutes

Serving Size: 1

Ingredients:

- 1 ripe banana
- 1/4 cup rolled oats
- 1/2 cup unsweetened almond milk
- 1 tablespoon honey (optional)

Instructions:

2. Blend all ingredients until smooth.

Nutritional Information (per serving):

- Calories: 180
- Protein: 4g

- Sodium: 80mg
- Potassium: 210mg
- Phosphorus: 80mg

Creamy Peach Smoothie

Prep Time: 5 minutes

Serving Size: 1

Ingredients:

- 1 ripe peach, pitted and chopped
- 1/2 cup plain Greek yogurt (low-fat)
- 1/2 cup unsweetened almond milk
- 1/4 teaspoon vanilla extract

Instructions:

1. Blend all ingredients until smooth.

Nutritional Information (per serving):

- Calories: 140
- Protein: 8g
- Sodium: 90mg
- Potassium: 220mg
- Phosphorus: 140mg

Carrot Cake Smoothie

Prep Time: 5 minutes

Serving Siz: 1

Ingredients:

- 1/2 cup shredded carrots
- 1/2 cup unsweetened coconut milk
- 1/4 cup Greek yogurt (low-fat)
- 1 tablespoon maple syrup
- 1/4 teaspoon ground cinnamon

Instructions:

1. Blend all ingredients until smooth.

Nutritional Information (per serving):

- Calories: 150
- Protein: 5g
- Sodium: 120mg
- Potassium: 260mg
- Phosphorus: 100mg

Chocolate Banana Protein Smoothie

Prep Time: 5 minutes

Serving Size: 1

Ingredients:

- 1 ripe banana
- 1 tablespoon cocoa powder
- 1/2 cup unsweetened almond milk

- 1 scoop vanilla protein powder (low-potassium)

Instructions:

1. Blend all ingredients until smooth.

Nutritional Information (per serving):

- Calories: 220
- Protein: 20g
- Sodium: 150mg
- Potassium: 300mg
- Phosphorus: 200mg

Coconut Berry Smoothie

Prep Time: 5 minutes

Serving Size: 1

Ingredients:

- 1/2 cup mixed berries (strawberries, blueberries, raspberries)
- 1/2 cup unsweetened coconut milk
- 1/4 cup plain Greek yogurt (low-fat)
- 1 tablespoon shredded coconut

Instructions:

1. Blend all ingredients until smooth.

Nutritional Information (per serving):

- Calories: 140

- Protein: 5g
- Sodium: 90mg
- Potassium: 180mg
- Phosphorus: 100mg

Vanilla Almond Smoothie

Prep Time: 5 minutes

Serving Size: 1

Ingredients:

- 1/2 cup unsweetened almond milk
- 1/2 cup plain Greek yogurt (low-fat)
- 1 tablespoon almond butter
- 1/4 teaspoon vanilla extract

Instructions:

1. Blend all ingredients until smooth.

Nutritional Information (per serving):

- Calories: 160
- Protein: 12g
- Sodium: 80mg
- Potassium: 180mg
- Phosphorus: 100mg

Minty Watermelon Smoothie

Prep Time: 5 minutes

Serving Size: 1

Ingredients:

- 1 cup diced watermelon
- 1/4 cup fresh mint leaves
- 1/2 cup unsweetened coconut water
- 1/4 cup plain Greek yogurt (low-fat)

Instructions:

1. Blend all ingredients until smooth.

Nutritional Information (per serving):

- Calories: 100
- Protein: 4g
- Sodium: 60mg
- Potassium: 200mg
- Phosphorus: 80mg

CHAPTER SIX:
30 DAYS MEAL PLAN

Day 1:

- Breakfast: Banana Oat Smoothie
- Snack: Carrot Sticks with Hummus
- Lunch: Grilled Chicken Salad with Mixed Greens and Lemon Vinaigrette
- Snack: Greek Yogurt with Sliced Peaches
- Dinner: Baked Salmon with Asparagus and Quinoa

Day 2:

- Breakfast: Berry Blast Smoothie
- Snack: Apple Slices with Almond Butter
- Lunch: Turkey and Avocado Wrap with Lettuce and Tomato
- Snack: Rice Cake with Cream Cheese and Cucumber Slices
- Dinner: Stir-fried tofu with Broccoli and Brown Rice

Day 3:

- Breakfast: Green Goddess Smoothie
- Snack: Greek Yogurt with Granola and Berries
- Lunch: Quinoa Salad with Chickpeas, Cucumber, and Feta Cheese
- Snack: Celery Sticks with Peanut Butter
- Dinner: Grilled Shrimp Skewers with Zucchini Noodles and Marinara Sauce

Day 4:

- Breakfast: Tropical Paradise Smoothie
- Snack: Mixed Nuts (unsalted)
- Lunch: Caprese Salad with Tomato, Mozzarella, and Basil
- Snack: Cottage Cheese with Pineapple Chunks
- Dinner: Baked Chicken Breast with Steamed Green Beans and Cauliflower Mash

Day 5:

- Breakfast: Creamy Peach Smoothie
- Snack: Rice Cake with Avocado and Cherry Tomatoes
- Lunch: Lentil Soup with Spinach and Carrots
- Snack: Orange Slices
- Dinner: Turkey Meatballs with Marinara Sauce over Spaghetti Squash

Day 6:

- Breakfast: Carrot Cake Smoothie
- Snack: Cucumber Slices with Hummus
- Lunch: Grilled Vegetable Wrap with Feta Cheese
- Snack: Almond Butter and Banana Slices on Whole Wheat Crackers
- Dinner: Baked Cod with Roasted Brussels Sprouts and Quinoa

Day 7:

- Breakfast: Chocolate Banana Protein Smoothie
- Snack: Greek Yogurt with Sliced Strawberries
- Lunch: Spinach Salad with Grilled Chicken, Strawberries, and Balsamic Vinaigrette
- Snack: Baby Carrots with Ranch Dressing (low-sodium)
- Dinner: Vegetable Stir-Fry with Tofu and Brown Rice

Day 8:

- Breakfast: Coconut Berry Smoothie
- Snack: Mixed Berries (strawberries, blueberries, raspberries)
- Lunch: Turkey and Cranberry Sandwich on Whole Wheat Bread
- Snack: Cottage Cheese with Sliced Kiwi
- Dinner: Baked Eggplant Parmesan with Mixed Green Salad

Day 9:

- Breakfast: Vanilla Almond Smoothie
- Snack: Apple Slices with Peanut Butter
- Lunch: Mediterranean Chickpea Salad with Feta Cheese and Lemon Herb Dressing
- Snack: Greek Yogurt with Granola and Honey
- Dinner: Grilled Steak with Roasted Vegetables and Quinoa

Day 10:

- Breakfast: Minty Watermelon Smoothie
- Snack: Mixed Nuts (unsalted)
- Lunch: Veggie Wrap with Hummus and Sliced Bell Peppers
- Snack: Celery Sticks with Cream Cheese
- Dinner: Baked Halibut with Steamed Asparagus and Wild Rice

Day 11:

- Breakfast: Mixed Berry Smoothie Bowl with Granola and Chia Seeds
- Snack: Sliced Cucumber with Tzatziki Sauce
- Lunch: Turkey and Avocado Wrap with Lettuce and Tomato
- Snack: Rice Cake with Almond Butter and Banana Slices
- Dinner: Grilled Lemon Herb Chicken with Roasted Cauliflower and Brown Rice

Day 12:

- Breakfast: Green Goddess Smoothie with Spinach, Kale, and Pineapple
- Snack: Greek Yogurt with Mixed Berries and a Drizzle of Honey
- Lunch: Quinoa Salad with Black Beans, Corn, Cherry Tomatoes, and Lime Vinaigrette
- Snack: Carrot Sticks with Hummus
- Dinner: Baked Cod with Roasted Brussels Sprouts and Quinoa

Day 13:

- Breakfast: Mango Coconut Chia Pudding
- Snack: Apple Slices with Almond Butter
- Lunch: Grilled Vegetable Panini with Mozzarella Cheese on Whole Wheat Bread
- Snack: Greek Yogurt with Sliced Strawberries and a Sprinkle of Granola
- Dinner: Baked Turkey Meatballs with Marinara Sauce over Zucchini Noodles

Day 14:

- Breakfast: Banana Oatmeal Pancakes with Maple Syrup
- Snack: Mixed Nuts (unsalted)
- Lunch: Spinach and Feta Stuffed Chicken Breast with Steamed Green Beans
- Snack: Cottage Cheese with Pineapple Chunks
- Dinner: Lentil Soup with Spinach and Carrots served with Whole Grain Bread

Day 15:

- Breakfast: Blueberry Almond Butter Smoothie
- Snack: Rice Cake with Avocado and Tomato Slices
- Lunch: Greek Salad with Romaine Lettuce, Cucumber, Tomato, Feta Cheese, and Kalamata Olives
- Snack: Celery Sticks with Peanut Butter

- Dinner: Grilled Salmon with Lemon Dill Sauce, Roasted Asparagus, and Quinoa

Day 16:

- Breakfast: Peanut Butter Banana Smoothie with a Dash of Cinnamon
- Snack: Greek Yogurt with Sliced Peaches and a Drizzle of Agave Syrup
- Lunch: Turkey and Cranberry Wrap with Mixed Greens and Balsamic Vinaigrette
- Snack: Mixed Berries (strawberries, blueberries, raspberries)
- Dinner: Baked Chicken Thighs with Roasted Vegetables and Wild Rice

Day 17:

- Breakfast: Strawberry Banana Chia Seed Pudding
- Snack: Carrot Sticks with Hummus
- Lunch: Veggie and Hummus Wrap with Bell Peppers, Cucumber, and Baby Spinach
- Snack: Cottage Cheese with Sliced Kiwi
- Dinner: Grilled Shrimp Skewers with Quinoa Tabbouleh Salad

Day 18:

- Breakfast: Peach Raspberry Smoothie Bowl with Granola and Shredded Coconut
- Snack: Rice Cake with Almond Butter and Sliced Banana

- Lunch: Caprese Salad with Tomato, Mozzarella, Basil, and Balsamic Glaze
- Snack: Greek Yogurt with Mixed Berries and a Drizzle of Honey
- Dinner: Baked Eggplant Parmesan with Whole Wheat Spaghetti

Day 19:

- Breakfast: Mango Coconut Smoothie with Spinach and Kale
- Snack: Sliced Cucumber with Tzatziki Sauce
- Lunch: Quinoa and Black Bean Stuffed Bell Peppers with Avocado Slices
- Snack: Greek Yogurt with Sliced Strawberries and a Sprinkle of Granola
- Dinner: Grilled Lemon Herb Chicken with Steamed Broccoli and Brown Rice

Day 20:

- Breakfast: Blueberry Almond Smoothie Bowl with Almond Butter and Chia Seeds
- Snack: Mixed Nuts (unsalted)
- Lunch: Turkey and Avocado Wrap with Lettuce, Tomato, and Mustard
- Snack: Apple Slices with Peanut Butter
- Dinner: Baked Cod with Roasted Brussels Sprouts and Quinoa

Day 21:

- Breakfast: Mixed Berry Smoothie with Spinach and Greek Yogurt

- Snack: Carrot Sticks with Hummus
- Lunch: Greek Salad with Romaine Lettuce, Cucumber, Tomato, Olives, and Feta Cheese
- Snack: Cottage Cheese with Pineapple Chunks
- Dinner: Grilled Chicken Breast with Roasted Vegetables and Quinoa

Day 22:

- Breakfast: Banana Peanut Butter Smoothie with Oats and Honey
- Snack: Greek Yogurt with Mixed Berries and a Drizzle of Agave Syrup
- Lunch: Turkey and Cranberry Wrap with Mixed Greens and Balsamic Vinaigrette
- Snack: Rice Cake with Almond Butter and Sliced Banana
- Dinner: Baked Salmon with Asparagus and Wild Rice

Day 23:

- Breakfast: Mango Coconut Chia Pudding with Sliced Almonds
- Snack: Apple Slices with Peanut Butter
- Lunch: Quinoa Salad with Black Beans, Corn, Tomato, Avocado, and Lime Vinaigrette
- Snack: Mixed Nuts (unsalted)
- Dinner: Lentil Soup with Spinach and Carrots served with Whole Grain Bread

Day 24:

- Breakfast: Blueberry Almond Butter Smoothie with Spinach and Flaxseeds
- Snack: Sliced Cucumber with Tzatziki Sauce
- Lunch: Caprese Salad with Tomato, Mozzarella, Basil, and Balsamic Glaze
- Snack: Greek Yogurt with Sliced Strawberries and a Sprinkle of Granola
- Dinner: Grilled Lemon Herb Chicken with Steamed Broccoli and Brown Rice

Day 25:

- Breakfast: Peach Raspberry Smoothie Bowl with Granola and Coconut Flakes
- Snack: Rice Cake with Avocado and Tomato Slices
- Lunch: Turkey and Avocado Wrap with Lettuce, Cucumber, and Mustard
- Snack: Mixed Berries (strawberries, blueberries, raspberries)
- Dinner: Grilled Shrimp Skewers with Quinoa Tabbouleh Salad

Day 26:

- Breakfast: Peanut Butter Banana Smoothie with Cinnamon and Honey
- Snack: Greek Yogurt with Mixed Berries and a Drizzle of Honey

- Lunch: Veggie and Hummus Wrap with Bell Peppers, Cucumber, and Baby Spinach
- Snack: Carrot Sticks with Hummus
- Dinner: Baked Eggplant Parmesan with Whole Wheat Spaghetti

Day 27:

- Breakfast: Mango Coconut Smoothie with Kale and Chia Seeds
- Snack: Apple Slices with Almond Butter
- Lunch: Quinoa and Black Bean Stuffed Bell Peppers with Avocado Slices
- Snack: Greek Yogurt with Sliced Strawberries and a Sprinkle of Granola
- Dinner: Grilled Lemon Herb Chicken with Steamed Green Beans and Brown Rice

Day 28:

- Breakfast: Blueberry Almond Smoothie Bowl with Almond Butter and Chia Seeds
- Snack: Mixed Nuts (unsalted)
- Lunch: Turkey and Avocado Wrap with Lettuce, Tomato, and Mustard
- Snack: Rice Cake with Almond Butter and Sliced Banana
- Dinner: Baked Cod with Roasted Brussels Sprouts and Quinoa

Day 29:

- Breakfast: Mixed Berry Smoothie with Spinach and Greek Yogurt
- Snack: Carrot Sticks with Hummus
- Lunch: Greek Salad with Romaine Lettuce, Cucumber, Tomato, Olives, and Feta Cheese
- Snack: Cottage Cheese with Pineapple Chunks
- Dinner: Grilled Chicken Breast with Roasted Vegetables and Quinoa

Day 30:

- Breakfast: Banana Peanut Butter Smoothie with Oats and Honey
- Snack: Greek Yogurt with Mixed Berries and a Drizzle of Agave Syrup
- Lunch: Turkey and Cranberry Wrap with Mixed Greens and Balsamic Vinaigrette
- Snack: Rice Cake with Almond Butter and Sliced Banana
- Dinner: Baked Salmon with Asparagus and Wild Rice

CHAPTER SEVEN: MANAGING DIET OVER TIME

As individuals age, their nutritional needs and health conditions may evolve, necessitating adjustments to their diet. Properly managing these changes is crucial for maintaining optimal health and well-being. In this section, we'll explore the importance of adjusting the diet as health changes occur, providing practical tips and guidance for navigating these transitions.

Understanding the Need for Dietary Adjustments:

One of the key reasons for adjusting the diet as health changes is to accommodate the evolving nutritional requirements of the body. As individuals age, they may experience changes in metabolism, nutrient absorption, and overall health status. Certain medical conditions, such as diabetes, hypertension, or kidney disease, may also require dietary modifications to manage symptoms and optimize health outcomes.

For example, individuals with diabetes may need to monitor their carbohydrate intake more closely to manage blood sugar levels effectively. Similarly, those with hypertension may benefit from reducing sodium intake to help regulate blood pressure. In cases of kidney disease, limiting potassium and phosphorus intake becomes essential to prevent complications and maintain kidney function.

Moreover, aging often brings about changes in appetite, taste preferences, and chewing or swallowing abilities, which can further impact dietary habits. As a result, adapting the diet to meet these changing needs becomes imperative for promoting overall health and quality of life.

Practical Tips for Adjusting the Diet:

1. **Regular Health Monitoring:** Regular health check-ups and consultations with healthcare professionals are essential for assessing any changes in health status and nutritional needs. Monitoring key indicators such as blood pressure, blood sugar levels, kidney function, and nutrient levels can help identify any potential dietary adjustments that may be necessary.

2. **Individualized Approach:** Every individual's dietary needs and health conditions are unique, so it's crucial to tailor dietary adjustments to meet specific requirements. Consulting with a registered dietitian or nutritionist can provide personalized guidance and support in developing an appropriate eating plan based on individual health goals and preferences.

3. **Gradual Changes:** When making dietary adjustments, it's essential to implement changes gradually to allow for adaptation and minimize any potential discomfort or adverse effects. Slowly introducing new foods or modifying portion sizes can help ease the transition and promote long-term adherence to the new eating plan.

4. **Focus on Nutrient-Rich Foods:** Emphasizing nutrient-rich foods such as fruits, vegetables, whole grains, lean proteins, and healthy fats is essential for supporting overall health and well-being. These foods provide essential vitamins, minerals, antioxidants, and fiber, which are vital for maintaining optimal health and preventing chronic diseases.

5. **Hydration:** Adequate hydration is crucial for overall health, especially as individuals age. Encouraging regular intake of water and other hydrating fluids can help prevent dehydration, support digestion, and promote healthy kidney function.

6. **Mindful Eating:** Practicing mindful eating techniques, such as paying attention to hunger and fullness cues, savoring the flavors and textures of food, and avoiding distractions during meals, can help improve digestion, promote satiety, and prevent overeating.

7. **Physical Activity:** Incorporating regular physical activity into daily routine is essential for maintaining overall health and supporting metabolic function. Engaging in activities such as walking, swimming, or yoga can help improve cardiovascular health, muscle strength, and flexibility.

Long-term Monitoring of Potassium Levels

Maintaining optimal potassium levels is crucial for overall health and well-being, as this essential mineral plays a vital role in various physiological processes within the body. However, imbalances in potassium levels can have serious health consequences, ranging from muscle weakness and fatigue to irregular heart rhythms and even cardiac arrest. Therefore, long-term monitoring of potassium levels is essential for identifying any deviations from the norm and implementing appropriate interventions to prevent adverse health outcomes.

Understanding Potassium Balance:

Potassium is an electrolyte that plays a critical role in maintaining fluid balance, regulating blood pressure, supporting muscle contractions, and facilitating nerve function. The body tightly regulates potassium levels through a complex interplay of factors, including dietary intake, renal excretion, and cellular uptake. Under normal circumstances, the kidneys help maintain potassium balance by excreting excess potassium into the urine, while the gastrointestinal tract absorbs potassium from dietary sources as needed.

Factors Affecting Potassium Levels:

Several factors can influence potassium levels in the body, including dietary intake, kidney function, medications, and certain medical conditions. High-potassium foods such as bananas, oranges, tomatoes, potatoes, and leafy greens can contribute to increased potassium levels, while low-potassium diets or certain medications may lead to potassium depletion. Moreover, conditions such as chronic kidney disease, diabetes, heart failure, and adrenal insufficiency can impair potassium regulation, leading to hyperkalemia (high potassium levels) or hypokalemia (low potassium levels).

The Importance of Long-Term Monitoring:

Long-term monitoring of potassium levels is essential for individuals at risk of potassium imbalances, particularly those with underlying medical conditions or taking medications that may affect potassium metabolism. Routine monitoring allows healthcare providers to assess potassium levels over time, identify any trends or fluctuations, and intervene promptly if abnormalities are detected. Early detection and management of potassium imbalances can help prevent complications and optimize health outcomes.

Monitoring Methods:

Potassium levels can be measured through various laboratory tests, including blood tests, urine tests, and occasionally, sweat tests. The most common method for assessing potassium levels is through a blood test, which measures the concentration of potassium in the blood plasma. Normal potassium levels typically range from 3.5 to 5.0 millimoles per liter (mmol/L), although reference ranges may vary slightly between laboratories.

Blood tests for potassium may be ordered as part of routine health screenings, during evaluations for specific medical conditions, or in response to symptoms suggestive of potassium imbalances, such as weakness, fatigue, muscle cramps, or cardiac arrhythmias. Additionally, individuals with chronic medical conditions or those taking medications known to affect potassium levels may require more frequent monitoring to ensure optimal potassium balance.

Interpreting Potassium Levels:

Interpreting potassium levels requires careful consideration of various factors, including the individual's overall health status, medical history, dietary habits, medications, and other laboratory parameters. Both hyperkalemia and hypokalemia can have serious health implications, so it's essential to assess potassium levels in the context of the individual's clinical presentation and risk factors.

Hyperkalemia, characterized by elevated potassium levels above the normal range, can result from impaired renal function, excessive potassium intake, certain medications (such as potassium-sparing diuretics or angiotensin-converting enzyme inhibitors), or acute medical conditions such as tissue breakdown (rhabdomyolysis) or metabolic acidosis. Hypokalemia, on the other hand, occurs when potassium levels fall below the normal range and may be caused by factors such as inadequate dietary intake, excessive potassium loss (e.g., due to diuretic use or gastrointestinal disorders), or certain medical conditions such as hyperaldosteronism or renal tubular acidosis.

Clinical Implications and Interventions:

Depending on the severity and underlying cause of potassium imbalances, interventions may vary. In cases of mild to moderate hyperkalemia or hypokalemia, dietary modifications and adjustments to medications may be sufficient to restore potassium balance. This may involve reducing or increasing dietary potassium intake, discontinuing potassium supplements, adjusting medication dosages, or addressing underlying medical conditions contributing to potassium imbalances.

In more severe cases or those associated with acute symptoms or complications, more aggressive interventions may be necessary. For hyperkalemia, treatments may include administration of medications to promote potassium excretion (such as loop diuretics or potassium-binding resins), intravenous fluids with dextrose and insulin to shift potassium into cells, or dialysis in cases of renal failure. Conversely, hypokalemia may require oral or intravenous potassium supplementation, along with addressing any underlying causes contributing to potassium depletion.

Long-Term Management Strategies:

In addition to acute interventions, long-term management of potassium imbalances involves ongoing monitoring, lifestyle modifications, and adherence to treatment regimens. Individuals with chronic medical conditions or those at risk of recurrent potassium imbalances may benefit from regular follow-up appointments with healthcare providers to assess potassium levels, review medications, and adjust treatment plans as needed. Moreover, educating patients about the importance of dietary potassium intake, medication adherence, and early recognition of symptoms suggestive of potassium imbalances can empower them to take an active role in managing their health.

CHAPTER EIGHT: CONCLUSION

Throughout this comprehensive guide, we have embarked on a detailed exploration of the low-potassium diet, particularly tailored for seniors. Our journey began with an understanding of potassium's vital roles and the circumstances under which a low-potassium diet becomes necessary. We have covered the spectrum from the biochemical significance of potassium in the body to the critical medical reasons that may necessitate such a diet for older adults.

The intricacies of controlling potassium consumption in the elderly population have been made clear by our discussions. We discussed the many illnesses that older adults face and how closely they need to be watched for potassium imbalances, including heart problems, hypertension, and kidney disease. We emphasized the need for seniors and those who care for them to exercise caution since severely elevated potassium levels can present major health hazards.

Moreover, we tackled the practical aspects of implementing a low-potassium diet, providing a thorough guide on foods to prioritize and those to avoid. We broke down the often-overlooked importance of understanding food labels—a crucial skill for maintaining such a diet while navigating grocery aisles and menus effectively. The sections dedicated to detailed food lists, alongside creative and nourishing recipes for meals throughout the day, were crafted to ensure that maintaining a low-potassium diet never becomes a mundane chore but rather an enjoyable culinary venture.

We also talked about how important it is for healthcare professionals to manage a low-potassium diet in parallel. By adjusting the diet to each person's evolving health status, regular consultations guarantee that it stays safe and effective. We also took supplements into account and provided advice on how to maintain general health without lowering potassium levels.

As we wrap up this guide, it's important to stress the dynamic nature of dietary management. Adjusting one's diet as health changes and ensuring long-term monitoring of potassium levels are not just recommendations; they are integral to sustaining health and wellness in senior years. The strategies and insights provided here are meant to empower seniors and their caregivers with the knowledge and tools needed for successful diet management.

This guide is more than just a collection of nutritional advice—it is a beacon for those navigating the complexities of health in senior years. Embracing a low-potassium diet with the right knowledge, support, and culinary creativity can transform a necessity into a positive lifestyle change. Here's to finding joy in the journey toward sustained health and vitality through mindful eating and informed choices. May this guide serve as a trusted companion in your ongoing pursuit of wellness.

www.ingramcontent.com/pod-product-compliance
Lightning Source LLC
Chambersburg PA
CBHW050107230526
45470CB00004B/1721